C000163480

TEARS
BEHIND CLOSED DOORS

TEARS
BEHIND CLOSED DOORS

by

Diana Holmes

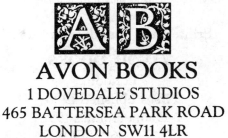

AVON BOOKS
1 DOVEDALE STUDIOS
465 BATTERSEA PARK ROAD
LONDON SW11 4LR

CARTOONS FOLLOWING PAGE 60:
© Margaret Ann Arkle

This book has been sold subject to the condition that it shall not, by
way of trade or otherwise, be lent, re-sold, hired out, photocopied or
held in any retrieval system, or otherwise circulated without the
publisher's consent in any form of binding or cover other than in
which this is published and without a similar condition including this
condition being imposed on the subsequent purchaser.

Printed and bound in the U.K.

Avon Books

London
First Published 1998
© Diana Holmes 1998
ISBN 1 86033 908 5

This book is dedicated to the Glory of God.

For patients, who have for a long time been intimidated, fobbed off, belittled and bullied by the medical profession because of the misinterpretation of thyroid function tests, then it is hoped, with the help of this book, they may regain the dignity that has been stripped from them.

Justice will always prevail in the end!

I have set the Lord always before me,
Because He is at my right hand,
I shall not be shaken.

Therefore my heart is glad and my glory rejoiceth:
My flesh also shall rest in hope.

Psalm 16: Verses 8-9

ACKNOWLEDGEMENTS

First and foremost a very big thank-you to my husband Norman for his support throughout my illness. For the constant understanding and encouragement during my years of research and campaign to raise the awareness of the misinterpretation of thyroid function tests.

Thank you for all the encouragement given by: Professor Nick Birch. Dr. Mike Wall – Director, Public Health Medicine, South Staffordshire, Dr. Peter Bourdillon, Department of Health, Dr. Heuck, World Health Organisation and Dr. Bill Reith, Royal College of General Practitioners.

To Sylvia, thank you for all her time and patience on the helpline.

Afshan Ahmed and Judith Davies for all their hard work in raising awareness of the problem of misinterpretation of thyroid function tests.

Thank you to Wendy Reid (journalist) and Evelyn Hood (author) for helping me to put my own personal story into order.

Malcolm Reid, thank you for the excellent articles in the *Glasgow Evening Times*.

To Alison Wick – Health Editor, *Woman* magazine. Thank you for all your time and effort and faith in the campaign.

I say to everyone who has submitted a story or poem. Thank you.

Thank you Dr. Peatfield for diagnosing me correctly in the first place.

My heartfelt thanks go out to Dr. Gordon Skinner, M.D. D.Sc. F.R.C.Path F.R.C.O.G., for his tenacity and commitment towards the campaign to raise awareness of the misinterpretation of thyroid function tests.

I would like to pay tribute to Caroline Hulme, who has for the last 13 years run a help-line for people suffering with thyroid conditions.

A special thank-you is due to Sean Ward, Chief Officer, Community Health Council, Wolverhampton, for his continued support.

Finally, a thank-you to Sir Patrick Cormack MP for his support and encouragement.

CONTENTS

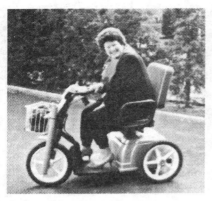

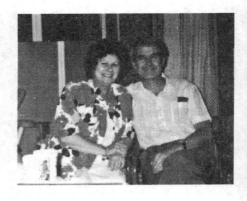

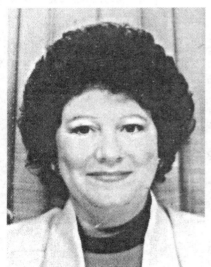

Compare these earlier photographs with the portrait of the 'new me' on the back of this book! This demonstrates the terrible and relentless physical debility which characterizes hypothyroidism, but it also shows that with carefully considered treatment we can all regain the vitality which, in the darkest periods of illness, we thought we had lost for ever. There is always hope!

This is the story of one of life's amazing survivors. It is the inspired account of a woman, who, from childhood, suffered emotional deprivation and physical illness, yet from a tender age, showed the remarkable will of mind, spirit and body that pulls through only the very few who have been to the brink and beyond.

It charts the course of an ordinary woman with extraordinary strength who survived a broken home, childhood polio, two broken marriages, the death of her beloved granddaughter and a crippling illness which she was to endure for twenty three years. She also brought up three children, struggling hard against the pain and debilitating effects of her illness.

However, despite the odds and fearing death, the inner spirit, which had driven her on through the gamut of tragedies which beset her life, triumphed and she proved everyone wrong.

She conquered her crippling illness, going against a medical establishment which had diagnosed her with six serious illnesses which had eventually confined her to a wheelchair.

Today, Diana Holmes, aged 55, has cast aside the shackles of ill health and has researched and found the reason why the medical profession missed her low thyroid disorder. She spends hours and hours every day in her search for more medical knowledge in order to prevent others going through the physical and emotional hell she had to endure. Her life's mission is to help others, both as informant with medical information which can improve their health, and as a spiritual shoulder to lean on to help them through the mire of their pitiful situation.

Here is Diana Holmes' story…it could so easily be yours.

WENDY REID
Journalist

i

It is rare that a member of the lay public makes significant contribution to any of the medical or physical sciences. This is not because they have insufficient knowledge but because there is a tendency among professionals to close ranks both socially and intellectually and refuse to admit truth if it does not arise from fellow professionals. There is no more glowing exception to this rule than is exemplified by the teachings of Mrs. Diana Holmes in this fascinating book *Tears Behind Closed Doors*.

Diana will forgive my suggestion that this is a second visitation in that until relatively recently and indeed (perforce) prior to laboratory testing there was no laboratory method of diagnosing hypothyroidism and the disease was diagnosed by the clinical features of the patient; indeed it would serve our younger colleagues well if they would read older text books which tend to give excellent details of the discriminatory features of the disease and well exemplified by hypothyroidism. As laboratory tests for hypothyroidism became more sophisticated there has been a gradual erosion of the pivotal role of clinical observation and an increasing reliance on laboratory estimation as a pivotal test of the diagnosis. This philosophy chooses to forget that these laboratory tests were originally evaluated by correlation with diagnoses which depended on clinical features and has reached its denouement in the present mindless deification of evidence-based medicine which is not evidence-based medicine but medicine based, usually, on laboratory evidence which is somehow considered more weighty than clinical observations in the nature of hypothermia, pulse rate or a subjective expression of symptomology by the patient; this misconception is motivated by the ever-increasing legal pressures where it is perceived that laboratory investigation will carry more weight in court than clinical observations, which is nonsense.

This unhappy situation condemns many patients — mainly women — to a wretched life, but hopefully will be redressed in the future. One of the major strategies towards this objective is patient empowerment, and this book by Diana Holmes is a major step in this direction. The book is beautifully written, anecdotal in content and motivated by Diana's personal experience of her diagnosis of hypothyroidism being missed for years, during which time she was given a series of other diagnoses including epilepsy, coeliac disease, polymyalgia rheumatica, depression, myalgic encephalomyelitis and myasthenia gravis. I trust my colleagues will not take her findings and her report as criticism of their professional competence but rather as a salutary message which will encourage dependence on clinical observations assisted by laboratory tests which are good servants but bad masters.

I cannot recommend this book too highly, particularly for my professional colleagues. We medical people are too pompous and arrogant; we mither about and hesitate to treat hypothyroid patients who have marginal or even normal thyroid chemistry while happily prescribing antidepressants and corticosteroid preparations which may well be justified but will almost never have any laboratory evidence of the patient's psychology or mood or the circulating level of steroid hormones, for example, in patients who are being treated for asthma; I am not suggesting that this is necessary but merely making a plea in deference to Diana's book for at least a more even-handed approach to pursuing the holy grail of evidence-based medicine.

G. R. B. S.
1998

I was a happy child, bright, bubbly, bursting with energy and most importantly, healthy. I had dreams of an exciting and wonderful future that are the right of every innocent child who trips along the path of life never expecting to falter.

At the age of eleven-and-a-half, I developed polio and in my mind, I had my first real battle with the medical establishment. My doctors wanted me to rest and not put any pressure on my leg, which was in a calliper. Needless to say, I did not do as I was told. If I had, I would most probably have still been in a wheel-chair. I consider having polio to be the first crack in the health network of my body and the emotional problems of the break-up of my parents' marriage when I was six years old, left me vulnerable emotionally too.

My teenage years culminated with my decision to become a nurse, but after a year, despite loving my career and the caring environment in which I had hoped to nurture others, my health was not at all that it should have been, although it was a mystery to me why I didn't have the energy or the mental resilience to cope with work.

I had always wanted to be a nurse from the time I was a little girl and after leaving school and trying a few other jobs, I took an entrance exam to train to be a S.R.N. (State Registered Nurse).

I was to complete one year. I scraped through the first year exams but found I just could not cope. If I had been on a split duty, I used to sleep until it was time to go on duty again. I was ashamed of this and never told anyone. Also, I was heartbroken not to be able to carry on with the training.

I married at the age of twenty and had two wonderful little girls, Julie and Tanya. My husband and I decided that, as we had been blessed with a healthy family, we would be content in the joy of our daughters and finish our family at that point. To that end, I had a coil fitted in the neck of my womb to prevent any further pregnancies.

That was to be the start of the nightmarish years which followed, as my health declined to such a state whereby I could only shuffle as exhaustion took over my body completely.

Over a period of twenty three years, I was misdiagnosed six times with serious diseases and treated for them. In the following chapters, I shall reveal how I overcame the misdiagnoses and how my life was to change when a private G.P. diagnosed me correctly with an underactive thyroid and made me the well woman I am today. My own G.P. had previously tested me for a low thyroid condition but the blood test result was returned "normal range", which according to my G.P., did not warrant treatment. Whereas the private G.P., regardless of the blood test result, prescribed thyroid replacement therapy and I became well.

I realised something was very wrong with present "clinical practice" carried out by the medical profession regarding thyroid function tests and I decided to investigate this area to try to discover where the problem lay.

The answer was in the interpretation of blood tests. I wrote a report and started a campaign to raise awareness of the problem.

From the onset the Department of Health and the World Health Organisation supported me in my endeavours.

For three years, I fought back against prejudice but I am now experiencing an increasing acceptance by the medical profession. I sent reference papers to thousands of patients who contacted me, and they in turn took these to their G.P. Many G.P.s took the information on board and acted upon it with the result that many hundreds of patients have regained their heath.

Dr. Gordon R.B. Skinner (MD., DSc., FRCPath,., FRCOG.) looked at my report eighteen months ago and agreed with my findings and subsequently has seen hundreds of patients who are suffering with hypothyroidism but with a "normal" blood test result. He has treated the majority of these patients and their health has improved significantly.

Thousands of people are caught up in the thyroid trap and these include M.E. sufferers. Years ago, Dr. Skinner realised that there may be a correlation between a low thyroid condition and some patients who suffer with M.E. and again, he has treated scores of these patients who are now in good health, which is very exciting.

Readers will be able to relate to my story and also to the other stories contributed by fellow sufferers.

In July 1997, I convened a meeting between Dr. Anthony Toft, President of the British Thyroid Association and Head of the Endocrine Unit of Edinburgh Royal Infirmary, Dr. Skinner and myself.   At the end of the meeting, Dr. Toft agreed to conduct a "clinical trial". This was more than we could have hoped for.   For three years, I had been aiming for this and now it was here.   The "trial" will be on-going for at least eighteen months to two years.

After reading my story in the *Glasgow Evening Times* Dr. E.H. McLaren, consultant physician at Stobhill N.H.S. Trust Hospital, will also be carrying out a double blind placebo controlled trial of thyroxine given to patients with symptoms of hypothyroidism and normal results of thyroid function tests.

The clinical trial, in this instance, will be a double blind trial, whereby some patients, who have a normal thyroid blood test result but yet experience many signs and symptoms of hypothyroidism, will be given thyroxine and some will be given a placebo. The person who is conducting the trial does not know who is given which.

The interpretation of thyroid function tests is the same world-wide and I am campaigning for a change in clinical practice re the interpretation of thyroid function tests. This book has been written to give comfort to those who have suffered and are now well and hope to those who are, as yet, still suffering.

D. H.
1998

CHAPTER ONE

OPERATION COIL

I froze! My G.P. had just given me the result of my pregnancy test – it was positive. There must be a mistake, I couldn't possibly be pregnant. I had had a coil fitted to the neck of my womb only three weeks ago and yet the doctor was telling me I was pregnant. He proceeded to examine me and then told me that I was at least three months pregnant.

That was to be the start of the nightmarish years which followed, resulting in ill-health that plagued me for the next twenty three years.

I had dreadful fears for the safety of my baby which was developing with that foreign body embedded in my womb. Although we had not planned on any more family, I rejoiced in the fact that I would have another child. These worries, that a new young life could be disfigured because of the coil, plagued me until the day my lovely son, Wayne, was born.

At a later date, I discovered that the consultant who had inserted the coil had written in his notes "womb bulky" and that alone should have alerted him to the fact that I could possibly be pregnant.

Following the birth of my son, my health deteriorated and I was found to be suffering from a womb infection which was blamed on the coil which was still inside me.

I attended a clinic twice a week for deep heat treatment for the infection, and while coping with my own health troubles, my son contracted whooping cough. I nursed him at home, tipping him upside down every half an hour to drain his lungs, both night and day, as I had been instructed. My maternal instincts for him fortunately overcame the exhaustion I was feeling.

1

On top of that, I still had to cope with everyday tasks, such as washing, ironing, cooking, cleaning and shopping.

My son's whooping cough cleared after six weeks, but I carried on attending the clinic for my health problems for another five months. When my son was twelve months old, I haemorrhaged badly and was taken into hospital for a "D & C" (dilation and curettage).

Unfortunately, this still didn't solve the problem and the surgeon asked if it might be better to have the coil removed surgically.

I returned home to consider this option but struggled on, still feeling unwell and eventually realised that I really didn't have any other option but to have the coil removed by operation.

The specialist was not at all surprised when I returned to see him. He arranged an admission to a hospital and explained he would try and remove the coil from the vagina but that if he couldn't he would have to operate.

It took medical staff five hours to bring me round from the anaesthetic. I felt so dizzy and disorientated and had trouble getting my words out, it was all very frightening.

The surgeon explained that he had had to open me up as he was afraid of rupturing my womb. He also confirmed that the coil had adhered itself to the wall of the womb and that I had, in effect, a double womb with a septum down the middle. I felt so ill and dizzy that this information was of no importance to me at the time.

Five weeks later, I was still in hospital and still feeling incredibly ill. Being told to pull myself together and get well for my three young children waiting at home was a constant message emanating from all quarters of the medical fraternity. I couldn't believe, in my naivety and misplaced awe of the medical profession, that in fact the doctors may be wrong and that my reaction to my situation was not a depressive one but a physical illness.

No one needed to remind me that I had a wonderful family at home waiting for a mother to nurture them, but they did not understand my pain. I could not walk too far without feeling dizzy, never mind look after three young children, a husband and a home. This seemed to be of no consequence to them.

The powers that be decided that I was becoming too institutionalised and in a situation which was not conducive to me forcing myself to accept my responsibilities and get on with life. Arrangements were made for my discharge.

I arrived home and my children looked so well, so beautiful and so perfect but the shining lights of my life were apprehensive of me as I had been away for what must have seemed an eternity to them.

Although I still felt unwell, I tried to programme my mind to think positively, telling myself this was only temporary and that I would get better. After all, I was home, life was good and it was only a matter of time before I became well.

Weeks dragged on into months and my health was still poor and the dreadful dizziness continued unabated. Trying to cope with my existence was a hard and lonely experience. Nevertheless, I still had to look after my husband and three children.

The inevitable happened, when, in desperation, I turned to my G.P., that standby diagnosis which has become the modern day cop-out of the medical profession was thrust upon me – "depression and anxiety".

Over the years of struggle that followed, if I had a pound for every so-called neurotic, depressed woman I have listened to and empathised with, I'd be a rich woman. As it is, the riches of good health which I have since acquired by searching for knowledge of my own health problems and my subsequent quest to help others in the same situation, far outweigh any monetary rewards that anyone could give me.

In my trusting way, I believed, to a certain extent, that if the professional said I was suffering from depression therefore I must be. But there was always an inner strength, a survival instinct that made me fight against

3

their compartmentalising of me as yet another woman with depression.

Despite taking tranquillisers and antidepressants, which my G.P. assured me would alleviate any dizziness, which he supposed was caused by anxiety, the situation actually became worse.

Growing marital problems forced me to start thinking about becoming independent. I returned to work with a view to making a life for myself and my children without a partner. It was a huge struggle but I did it and after ten years of marriage, I was on my own and providing for my family despite the fact that my health was getting worse.

Then there was a little chink of light over the months. I started to feel a little better. My health was still not good but it was better.

Two years later, I met someone and moved away to another area. We shared a home together for a while and then eventually married. After twelve months of marriage, my health started to decline and I became exhausted and dizzy. I also became so sleepy that it was almost like a sleeping sickness. I could sleep most of the day and night.

As well as all that, I was developing muscular aches and pains, with particular problems in my back. I was sent to an orthopaedic specialist who carried out blood tests but all these tests came back "in the normal range".

My most vivid memory of that specialist was the accusing way in which he told me: "Well, you haven't got M.S.," (multiple sclerosis). I reeled in shock, both at his attitude and the fact that I had not even been informed that he suspected M.S.

For my muscular aches and pains, he told me that I needed manipulation under anaesthetic. This treatment was duly carried out with the result that the spinal problems were relieved for a while.

On top of everything else, over the next few months, I developed stomach and bowel disorders. I suffered greatly from indigestion and belching and my stools (motions) were pale and smelly.

What was wrong with me? That question I was to pose many time over the next decade.

I was determined to try and overcome these problems. The G.P. had said, some time ago, that I was suffering from depression and needed to be kept busy. I got a job in a potato packing factory but hadn't been there long before I suffered the most dreadful fainting attack. If I had passed out completely it would have been better but I didn't. I was very frightened. The management decided to send me home by taxi. I realised that heavy physical work was beyond my capability and gave in my notice.

My G.P. was, once again, in a quandary and he decided to refer me to the orthopaedic specialist again. This consultation resulted in a diagnosis of coeliac disease.

I had never heard of it but the specialist explained that it is an allergy to the protein (gluten) in wheat and rye.

I was put on a strict gluten-free diet, which meant cutting out all wheat and rye flour. Anyone who suffers from this disease will understand the problems I was then about to encounter.

I was under the impression that flour was used to make things like bread, cakes, biscuits etc.; but my subsequent investigations taught me that it is also used in food items as diverse as stock cubes and ice cream.

Planning menus for such a diet is a time consuming occupation and shopping becomes laborious, as every label has to be checked for the forbidden ingredients.

I remember one dear soul, who'd obviously been observing my antics in the supermarket, saying chirpily, "Looking for calories, dear?"

"No," said I, in a disgruntled fashion, "Flour."

She went off bemused and muttering about the strange dietary habits of today's young folks.

My energy level still continued to be way, way below par, and dizziness varied in intensity depending on my activities. And now I had coeliac disease. The list of physical disorders was growing and that was not even including the mental and emotional problems of just

5

coping with life when your health is on a continuing downward spiral.

I was also beginning to experience the terrible frustration and loneliness of ill-health, which is something all who suffer from long term or debilitating illnesses must experience but they try to conceal it. One feels ashamed yet dare not admit it to others. The feelings of anger which also well up until they reach an intolerable overspill, are also a huge part in the draining process of your emotional well-being.

I often imagined that if I could put the dizziness, sleepiness and the awful way I felt on the table in front of my G.P., he would then see that I was not making up this horrible nightmare. My desperation to quantify my illness to him was immense, yet it was an impossible task for me to convey this to him in anything that would remotely resemble facts.

He was a doctor, not a miracle worker. Unfortunately, many of them see themselves as miracle workers and not doctors. Ironically, if their miracles go awry, it's your fault and not theirs.

I continued to exist from day to day, trying to do the best for my children. They never said but they must have wondered what was wrong with their mummy.

I suffered more of those dreadful fainting spells and again felt very frightened. Everything kept going black. Things would clear, then would go black again. This kept happening on and off for a couple of hours. My heart raced and it felt as though it was coming out of my chest. I experienced these feelings many, many times and sometimes they lasted for hours on end.

It was back to the G.P. and a visit to a neurologist followed.

The neurologist said that he wanted to carry out an E.E.G. (electro-encephalogram). This is to record brain activity traced by a graph. He didn't talk to me and tell me why he was going to do this and I was too shy to ask. At that stage, I was beginning to harbour thoughts that I might have a brain tumour.

I had to wait for tests, wait for results and still the suffering went on, this time with added worries of the fear of the unknown result.

On the day of the second appointment with the neurologist, I was extremely nervous but told myself that I had to be positive. That is easier said than done.

The bombshell diagnosis this time was…epilepsy!

I couldn't move; I couldn't open my mouth. I just remember sitting there in disbelief. The doctor was rattling on telling me something I didn't want to hear and I couldn't take it in. When my mind started to function, it began racing with questions about epilepsy. What did it mean? Would I have convulsions? What about medication.

I had seen convulsions in my nursing days and they were not pleasant. My heart always went out to people who suffered with this condition and now I was being told that I had the same illness.

On the journey home, my mind was in a turmoil but one of the few things I managed to remember was that I was to see my G.P. who would prescribe medication that I would have to take for the rest of my life.

I reasoned with myself that if medication was to halt the dreadful cycle of sleeping and dizziness, then it was a small price to pay for a return to good health.

I saw my G.P. the very next day but he was surprised at the diagnosis and refused to prescribe any medication until he had received a report from the consultant. I had no argument with that and inside, I desperately hoped that they had made a mistake and maybe it wasn't epilepsy after all. I told myself to be realistic and to stop clutching at straws.

My G.P. despite this, was sympathetic and understanding and at least I had the immense relief of professionals actually believing that my problems were now physical and not emotional.

Eventually, I was prescribed medication which made me feel worse then ever. I persevered for two weeks, then, being able to stand it no longer, made yet another appointment with the doctor.

Again, he was very kind but told me to persevere for a little while longer and to see him each week to monitor the situation.

I did this for a period of three months and by this time, my G.P. had reached his own conclusion.

He informed me that he didn't think I was suffering from epilepsy at all but he was still clueless as to what could be causing my symptoms.

You could have knocked me down with a feather but then I experienced a momentary wave of relief. However, although it wasn't epilepsy the mystery of my debilitating health was to continue.

Medication was ceased and I felt better because the side effects stopped, although I still had my original health problems.

The saga continued as did the pain. A trip to the surgery was becoming as routine as a trip to the shops, but instead of a shopping list I would be clutching a prescription, as if it were a panacea for all my ills. I was being fed a diet of tranquillisers and anti-depressants and I was too ill and by now, too scared, to do anything other than swallow the poisons which were being pumped in copious quantities into my system.

At that stage in my life, at the age of thirty six, I remember envying old age pensioners as they passed me in the street. Compared to me, they were full of life but I just seemed to be getting older and more ill as each year progressed.

Over the years, my second marriage had suffered and I decided to break away for the second time and try to lead an independent life with my children, this time vowing never to have another partner while my children were still living with me.

So, there was another move, a new start in another district, a new job, and just enough money to invest in a small, two-bedroomed house. Emotionally, I felt dreadful, with the guilt of another failed marriage behind me and the continuing upset that I had put my children through.

Despite my deteriorating health, I needed to keep working in order to bring up my children and I had very strict views about not taking money from the State.

At the office where I worked, I sometimes fell asleep and the guilt of that overwhelmed me, as did the humiliation, if other colleagues commented on it, albeit jokingly.

During that spell of office work, I developed muscular problems with my fingers and on occasions, could not even write as my fingers contorted into the most grotesque shapes.

Yet another appointment with the G.P. ensued, but as I had moved districts by that time, I joined another practice and unfolded my medical history to the new doctor. He decided the problem with my fingers could be Carpal Tunnel Syndrome and I was duly sent off to yet another specialist for yet another test.

The diagnosis this time was "a bit of arthritis", yet another complaint to add to this never-ending list of mysterious health problems.

As I looked back over my life, days and months of illness and anguish turned into years and the exhaustion by this time was more intolerable than I can bear to describe.

My children coped – because they had to – they just seemed to accept that this was how family life was and I marvel at the resilience of children. They coped and survived. So, thank God, have I.

As the arthritis worsened, a locum at the surgery seemed to think I could be suffering from polymyalgia rheumatica – a muscular disease – and she prescribed 30mg of steroids a day.

Gradually, I started to feel brighter and less exhausted and by the end of two weeks, I actually began to feel good – a feeling that had been alien to me for so long. A month later, I felt better than I had in years with more energy in my forties than in my thirties.

However, this well-being was short-lived and when the locum left, my original G.P. refused to continue the treatment as he disagreed with the diagnosis.

Many years later, when I had access to my medical records, I was horrified to read that the G.P. in question felt I had manipulated the locum into prescribing steroids. At that time, I had never even heard of polymyalgia, let alone known what medication was needed. This was, indeed, another example of the paradox of what is termed the "caring profession".

It was back to square one and all my symptoms which had improved dramatically on the medication, swiftly returned – dizzy spells, exhaustion, aches and pains. Need I go on?

I remembered how difficult it was even to shop for the family as I couldn't carry a shopping bag without ending up in a state of total exhaustion. Collapsing on to a chair after each outing to the shops was the norm but even in that dreadful state, I still had the fight within me that refused to accept that this was my life ad infinitum. The medical profession would have to listen and with a renewed determination and conviction that there was an answer just waiting to be found, another trip was made back to the surgery.

The trouble with observations, rather than facts, in a patient's medical notes is that whenever a new doctor reads them, he is coloured by another professional's personal view of the situation.

I had been labelled a neurotic and a manipulator; I was neither. I was a very sick woman in need of expert help, yet no one was prepared to acknowledge it and give me the expertise I so desperately needed in order to give me back my life. I felt anger and frustration at being robbed of a good quality of life.

The trip to the surgery ended up with my health troubles being diagnosed as "psychological". When you are feeling so awful and ill to the brink of collapse, you grasp at any helping hand that is offered, even if, with the best intent, it is the wrong one.

I had been diagnosed with spondylitis in my neck many years before and as a platitude, my G.P. even suggested the spondylitis in my neck could have caused me to be unduly anxious about my health. I was not the only one grasping at straws!

As I looked over the last thirteen years – since my operation when I was twenty eight years old – there were not many times when I felt that my quality of life was good. There were spells when I felt better but those periods didn't last long, maybe a few months in total. Like a fool who grasps at gold, when I did feel better, I threw myself into life full-tilt but it always ended in another deterioration in health. It was a vicious circle that had to be broken. I didn't know how or when that re-direction would happen, or even more frightening, if it would happen at all.

A weak acceptance that I had a psychological problem led me to the doors of a psychologist and like a lamb to the proverbial slaughter I went along.

At that time, I'll admit to being depressed. I defy anyone who had a history of crippling health like mine not to be depressed in that situation.

The psychologist was kind and I cried many tears, expressing my innermost hurt and laying before her the external pains of the exhaustion I was suffering.

She began digging into my past, possibly in a bid to find other reasons which could have caused my depression but by the third visit she questioned whether I was gaining any benefit from these sessions. In her professional opinion, I was a well adjusted individual and she suggested that the sessions be discontinued.

That psychologist did more for me than she will ever know. She listened to me and she heard what I had to say.

It is so painfully true that many who profess to listen, just will not hear.

My mum died in 1982. She had been suffering from cancer of the womb and bowel. Shortly before she died, it was decided that she should stay with my sister, Penny, for her last days. I asked my eldest daughter, Julie (she had left home to set up on her own), if she would come home and take care of Tanya and Wayne in order that I could be with mum. My two sisters Penny and Liz, my brother Tony and myself stayed with mum and cared for her until she died.

Grieving for mum and the continuous cycle of pressure at home and at work, led to yet another deterioration in my health and I feared for the future.

Shortly after mum died, the company doctor at work decided that due to my ill health I was to be invalided out. He put my ill-health down to the spondylitis of the spine that had been diagnosed earlier. This in turn forced me to accept invalidity payments from the Department of Health and Social Security. I was not happy with this situation at all.

CHAPTER TWO

LOVE COMES IN

My son left school and gained employment some thirty miles away from home and had to move districts. He was the last of my children to leave and it was hard. I never thought that I would grieve because my children left home but I did.

I decided to sell my house and buy a mobile home to greatly reduce my outgoings.

Somebody I had met years earlier came back into my life and we became very close. He asked me if I would like to live with him in the Midlands. I agreed and one year later we were married. Norman is my beloved husband of eleven years and if anyone deserves a medal he does. His love, patience and protection over the years and his prayers for me to regain my health have been constant.

Despite finding a wonderful partner and managing to sustain a fulfilling relationship, notwithstanding my failing health, I felt everyone out there was living while I was just existing.

A few people judged me unfairly and told me I looked fine to them but they did not know all the facts. I was to learn, in the future, that even when people were in receipt of all the facts they still made unfair judgements.

While I was still in Cheshire, I took up art and became interested in painting. I couldn't paint for long spells but it was very rewarding. Holding a pencil sometimes caused my hands to contort into the most awful cramps. A paintbrush was different as I didn't have to hold it so hard. If I held it gently, I could still make it do what I wanted it to. Art, for me, was my saving grace at that time in my life and I managed to sell a few paintings which helped with the bills.

In 1988, I was sent to see a general physician at a hospital in the Midlands where I then lived. At this time I was still on a gluten-free diet. I had started to suffer with digestive upsets and an endoscopy under general anaesthetic was suggested. With this minor operation, an endoscope is inserted into the digestive track. It has a small camera on the end of it which allows the physician to locate any problems.

The physician who performed this operation subsequently told me that he was sure that I was not suffering from coeliac disease.

How many more times was I to be labelled with a disease, treated for it and then told I was not suffering from it? For eleven years I had been on a coeliac diet. Anyone suffering from it knows the frustration of its limitations. Those eleven years were erased with one sentence as the physician wrote in my notes, "Coeliac disease is not present."

By 1989, it was thought that I had the condition M.E. A blood sample was sent to London to Professor Mowbray and the result determined that an entero virus was present in my blood. I had had polio when I was aged eleven years, so that could have accounted for it and the condition of M.E. certainly fitted in with the way I was feeling. I had many more symptoms by that time including poor concentration and a sluggish memory.

So let's look at M.E. M.E. stands for "myalgic" (which relates to the muscles), "encephalo" (to the brain) and "mylitis" (inflammation of the spinal cord).

Norman and I decided to attend an M.E. meeting in Halesowen, to find out more about this disease. We drew up outside the hall where the meeting was to take place and I looked aghast at the steps up to the entrance. Steps had been a problem for a long time and we moved from a house to a bungalow because of this. However, we had come quite a long way and I was determined to go in. It took a while but with my husband's help I made it. Once inside, there were two more flights to climb and this meeting was for people with M.E.!! Nobody seemed to be having the difficulty that I was. Tears stung my eyes as I looked at Norman. He put his arm in mine and helped me up each step. At the end of the meeting, neither Norman nor I were fully convinced that I had M.E.!

In October 1990, we made a trip to see my brother Tony and sister-in-law Chris in Aberdeen. It was along journey, with lots to see and yet, because of my exhaustion, I could not keep my eyes open. I did see flashes of the countryside in between sleeping and realised how truly beautiful Scotland was in the autumn.

We stayed with Tony for a few days and I remember trying to cope with a disturbing cough. Upon leaving Aberdeen for the homeward journey, we had not gone far when I felt my chest tighten and I started to wheeze. Norman stopped the car and I tried to tell him what was wrong in between wheezes. As it got worse, I felt I needed a doctor. I could hardly breathe.

We stopped at a beautiful little village called Ballater and spotted a medical centre. We didn't have long before we were ushered into a room where we saw a lady G.P. She was most kind and listened to my chest and diagnosed asthma. She proceeded to show me how to use an inhaler that she had taken out of its box. This was all going too fast. Now I said she was kind and I meant it; but is it possible, when a doctor tells you that you have a serious disease, before they go launching off into a dialogue, they give you some time to adjust? I now added asthma to my growing list of ailments.

In November 1990, my condition became very much worse. Exhaustion was with me all the time, slowly torturing me like a never-ending drip of water which would soon turn into a deluge, under which I felt I would surely drown.

Upon waking, my head always felt muzzy, as if I were constantly in a fog and the sleep I experienced seemed like the sleep of the dead. Creases etched into my face and body. I slept so soundly and completely, as if I were a motionless body in a coma.

The colour of my skin was changing into an insipid grey pallor and becoming even drier and my nails were so brittle. In truth, I felt and looked like a walking corpse.

Even though I felt so ill, I always applied my make-up. I remember one time, with a temperature of 104 degrees Fahrenheit, I walked along a long hospital corridor with my full make-up on. I collapsed once I got to the ward but that is hardly the point.

My weight had increased from 9½ stone to 11½ stone and my voice had become hoarse and talking for any length of time made it worse. My movements were slow and awkward and my face was puffy.

My G.P. referred me to yet another consultant.

Another waiting room, another hospital. I am sure that there is more to life than this!

We were ushered in to the doctor's room. Undressed in my bra and pants, I lay on the couch. How many times had I done this, waiting for a doctor to come and examine me? I hated it, yes I hated it. Tears started to well up in my eyes. I must not cry, please God help me not to cry. I am quite a private person and I find no pleasure in repeatedly divulging my history to the medical profession.

That physician gave me the most thorough examination I have ever had to this day and took blood samples to do a few tests.

Another appointment followed and the physician said that he would like to carry out a "tensilon test", which would help him make a diagnosis. I didn't feel that I had much choice. He said that if the test proved positive that for a few minutes, I would feel better all round. The syringe was prepared and a solution was injected into my arm. Suddenly my eyes did not feel heavy any more, I could open them wide. I turned over on the couch, to my surprise, so easily, that I kept turning over and over. I soon tired of that and swung my legs to the floor.

16

I asked, "Could we go for a walk in the corridor?" The doctor agreed. I couldn't believe how fast I started to walk. I then noticed the doors through to the stairs, I went through the doors and took the stairs three at a time and cleared three flights in record time. The doctor then said that we must make our way back to his consulting room. I hadn't been in there long before I felt myself returning to the same state of lethargy that was with me when I first entered the room. I felt dreadful. Whatever it was had made me feel so good and yet it was so short-lived.

Two and a half years hence, I was to question the validity of this test.

The consultant told me that the results of the test indicated a disease called myasthenia gravis, which is a grave, progressive muscle disease. I did not move, I just sat there staring at him. My mind was trying to adjust to what he had said. Did he say a progressive muscle disease? Did that mean I was going to die soon? I blurted out, "What shall I do?" He started to talk to me and assured me that I was not about to die as the condition could be treated with medication. He prescribed steroids and mestinon tablets. My head was reeling!

Initially, the medication made me feel better but at a later date I put that down to the steroids. I had been diagnosed with myasthenia gravis in the November of 1990 and after Christmas, I had a troublesome cough and was wheezing very badly, even with inhalers. My G.P. stated that it was due to the myasthenia. The consultant who had diagnosed the myasthenia saw me in February and said I had a chest infection and took me into hospital. I was given oxygen, put on to an ever higher dose of steroids and every four hours the physiotherapist came and pummelled my back. It took twelve days, on massive doses of antibiotics, to clear the infection.

During the course of all this treatment, I was sent for another X-ray and as I found it impossible to walk more than a few paces, a wheel-chair was ordered for me.

The amount of medication I was on was extremely disturbing to me. I was on high doses of antibiotics, steroids and mestinon. I had been experiencing the most horrific cramps in my neck, back, hands and legs but the most frightening were in the neck as I thought I might choke. One day, the cramps in my legs were so bad that I cried out with pain. It was like being in labour all over again. I was in this state for hours. I cried out to God to help me! The nursing staff tried everything they could think of to relieve the pain. I was given quinine which helped a little. Eventually the cramps subsided. The infection cleared and I returned home to make the most of the quality of life I had left.

Positiveness is inherent in my nature and I had already realised that life, for me, from now on was going to be very different. I could no longer do the housework and needed help with the heavy cleaning and ironing. This was mentally hard for me and I began to feel guilty. It took some time to come to terms with the fact that somebody else was cleaning my home. Many people, who are ill, experience these feelings and it is a form of release to talk about it with others.

I started to look at what my life would consist of. I loved my husband and enjoyed cooking for him and although I could not see to many things, I could organise the household. I still painted and that brought in a few pennies. I attended church, which was fifty yards away from my doorstep and I began to see the positive side of my life instead of the negative side.

My condition became worse and Norman said that he would like to buy me a motorised wheel-chair. I fought against this idea at the beginning but as time went by I gave in. The buggy, I affectionately called "Bugsy", gave me an independence, which before I could only dream about. Previously I had to wait for someone to take me in the car if I wanted to go out, now the joy of being able to go out on my own was wonderful.

I found a new friend, she was suffering from cerebella-ataxia, this condition causes lack of co-ordination of movement. We travelled the village together in our buggies and stopped for coffee at "Flappers", the local coffee shop. We laughed or smiled together (laughing hurt my head).

However, there came a time when I could no longer use the buggy, because I did not have the strength to pull the lever to activate the forward motion.

I reached a stage whereby I did not have the energy to go out and I had become incontinent of both bowel and bladder. I felt the medication for the myasthenia was killing me.

Norman and I visited the Radcliffe Infirmary in Oxford, to see a consultant who specialised in myasthenia gravis. Tests were done and we were given the verdict. The consultant said that, in his opinion, I was not suffering from myasthenia gravis. My mouth gaped in incredulity. How many more times was I to be labelled with a disease, only to find out, after years of treatment, that I hadn't got it. On the way home, I cried with relief but also I felt very angry with the medical profession. I was slowly losing patience and respect for the establishment. Six misdiagnoses in one lifetime is enough for anyone.

I had been treated for myasthenia gravis for two-and-a-half years.

I asked my G.P. if he would help me to come off the medication for myasthenia gravis. He readily agreed. He then proceeded to tell me that he didn't believe that I had the condition!

After a few weeks, I began to feel a little better as the side effects from the drugs began to wear off. I came off the steroid medication very, very slowly but my health deteriorated and the anxiety I felt was frightening. I began to experience strong palpitations (i.e. the heart starts beating faster and jumping around in your chest).

CHAPTER THREE

LIGHT AT THE END OF THE TUNNEL

It was at this stage in my life that I turned to God. My Faith in God, since February 1991, has gone from strength to strength. I know now that had I not suffered in the way that I did, I would not have been able to apply myself to the work that I became involved in. That was to start in 1994.

In 1993, somebody said to me, "Have you got a thyroid problem?" I said, "I don't know." Still, it was worth asking my G.P. He readily agreed to send off a blood sample to test for thyroid function. I know he was almost as frustrated as I was because he couldn't find out what was wrong with me. The blood test for thyroid function went off to the laboratory. I had done some research in the library before going to the doctor's and discovered that thyroid problems could be easily treated, enabling sufferers to lead normal lives.

I began to hope that I had thyroid trouble but my hopes of living a normal life were dashed. The result of my blood test was returned "in the normal range". I felt so much despair and by now was badly depressed. Who wouldn't be after all that I had been through?

Norman was made redundant in 1993, which hit him hard, as it would anyone. At fifty-three years of age he was not going to find it easy to obtain employment again. So many people we knew were redundant. We decided to go away for the winter of '93/'94 to Spain and Portugal. We had been told it was much cheaper to live out there in the winter months. We bought a motor home and set off for the south on October 1st, 1993. The journey down to Portugal was horrific and very frightening. The motor home snaked across the roads because the dealer we bought the motor home from had not put the correct pressure in the tyres and we were inexperienced with this large vehicle. The weather was the worst Europe had seen for a long time. By the time we reached Portugal, I was in a very nervous, anxious state.

We returned home in April 1994 with me in very poor health. We had thought that the sun may have been good for me. My health had declined until I could only walk a few paces. Norman had to take over all household duties and I just lay on the settee.

Whatever this illness was it had progressed. I was beginning to think that I was losing my mind because it had started to play tricks on me. One day, while watching the T.V., I turned to Norman and his face took on the look of my mother, who had died many years earlier. It frightened me and I turned away. Spider phobias and hallucinations were to haunt me for a long while. I used to love speed in a car. Not anymore. Now I was afraid to travel in a car. I didn't like being shut up in a small room such as the toilet. Having a shower terrified me. The spray from the shower felt like needles piercing my skin.

Before I had been retired from work, I had taken out a Permanent Health Scheme to cover me in case of illness, never thinking that I would be retired from work because of ill-health.

The policy was sold on, from one company to another, until it was bought by a well-known company. I continued to receive payments from this company, under the terms of the policy, until one day they informed me that I was to be sent for a dynatron test. This I was told, would show up any problem with my muscles. I welcomed this although not the journey to London. The test was horrid and very painful. The dynatron test comprised pulling various limbs against a tensioned frame, the results of which are recorded on a computer. I was unable to complete the tests due to pain and fatigue.

We had travelled down by train and on the return journey I was very ill. The pains in my back and the exhaustion were awful. The steward said, "Would you like some ice packs?" I said, "Yes, please." He said he thought that I would feel more comfortable in the first class compartment and so took us along. At the end of the journey we thanked him very much for his kindness.

I attended the clinic in London for the dynatron test on the 23rd May, 1994.

The letter my doctor received from Unum is set out below.

"You may recall that we were in correspondence about this patient of yours last year. You will know that we have not been convinced about her disability for some little time and we therefore arranged an independent orthopaedic examination and a dynatron assessment in London. Our examiner was a distinguished teaching hospital orthopaedic surgeon.

"The conclusion is that there is no organic abnormality. Her symptoms are totally out of proportion to any objective evidence that there is and the gross variability in her response to the dynatron examination is a good demonstration that she was exerting volitional control over the examination.

"Our feeling, therefore, is that she is indeed fit to pursue her insured occupation and further benefit will not be paid."

If I were exerting volitional control over the examination as they suggested this surely makes a nonsense of the dynatron test. The patient, as I see it, is in a no win situation. They accused me of cheating the machine and of this I stand innocent before my God.

Can you imagine how I felt after I read that letter? The horrors of whatever it was I was suffering from were bad enough without being kicked, punched and kicked again while I was down. The stress that the dynatron test and the letter caused was indescribable and made my condition worse.

22

I have since been told by an independent Insurance Adviser that this 'rejection' is a common ploy of some Health Insurance companies.

I am hurting – I just shuffle along – I can't go any faster – when will the pain go away? – my body is so heavy – I am so exhausted but I must push on – Oh dear God please help me!

A few days after that event in London, my friend June said she was sure I had a thyroid problem and that there was a private doctor who would see me without a referral from my own G.P. I remarked to her, "I don't want another disease." Anyway, I had already been tested for the condition, without a positive result. June gave me a list of signs and symptoms to look at. These I put to one side.

Still my condition became worse. In the end I forced myself to read through the signs and symptoms and a slow realisation dawned on me. I was suffering from most of the signs and symptoms that were listed. Even the books from the library were not as clearly defined. Something else on the information; it stated that the blood tests were not specific enough. What did that mean?

I showed the signs and symptoms to Norman, who immediately brought me down to earth and reminded me that many times illnesses had been diagnosed, and then discounted, and who is to say that this was going to be any different? He was just warning me to be cautious. Nevertheless, we made an appointment to see the private G.P. Was this to be another blind alley or an open door to health?

I had a week to wait until I saw the private G.P. When there is hope on the horizon, patience goes out of the window and you want to be better yesterday. I made an appointment with my own G.P. to obtain his blessing, which he gave readily.

On the way to the private G.P. in Surrey, I felt a wonderful peace fill my soul. I knew that God was with me and with His grace, whatever was before me I could handle. Norman was quiet and thoughtful as we set out. What I had done to deserve Norman I will never know.

I do not remember the journey: I slept most of the way.

The words, "Well, Mrs. Holmes, you really are a deserving case," will ring in my ears forever. "Not only are you suffering from hypothyroidism (underactive thyroid) but also adrenal exhaustion," the doctor confirmed. Inside, instinctively I knew he was right. He prescribed medication and after collection from his dispensary we made our way home. Again, I slept most of the way.

I started the medication straight away. Two weeks went by and there was a slight improvement, my head cleared and some of the heaviness had gone out of my limbs, although I was still in a lot of pain. After the third week I was brighter mentally. This was something I had not experienced for a long time. One thing I will remember for a long while to come was being able to let the bath water run down my chest without it hurting. I noticed that my feet, bottom and hands had started to warm up. They had always been so cold before.

The dizziness left me! After all those years!

After two months, my skin and nails were better and my hands didn't tingle as much as before. After three months, I was able to go for a short walk. I still had to take it easy as I became very breathless. I cannot begin to tell you of the excitement I felt. After six months of treatment I could walk a mile. This was a miracle!

Because my head had cleared, I could laugh again without it hurting and laughter is such a joyful experience when it does not hurt your head to do it. My slurred speech cleared up and my voice was no longer hoarse. Scores of times, I had made mention to the doctors that my voice was so different from what it had been years ago.

Amazing things were happening to me. My pubic hair had started to grow again (so, losing one's pubic hair is not a pre-requisite for growing older) and my eyebrows. My ankles were no longer swollen. The puffiness around my eyes and face had gone.

During my years of illness and despair, my weight had shot up to 12st. 5lbs. I lost 9lbs in weight, without dieting, which brought my weight down to 11 stone 10 lbs.

The hearing sensitivity had cleared up. I had previously reached a stage whereby I could not stand noises of any kind. Even people speaking normally sounded as if they were shouting. I remember being very suspicious of everybody, even suspicious of my wonderful husband. That had all abated now. The hallucinations, noises and voices in the head had gone. I could now swallow without difficulty and I didn't have those choking fits over food and drink. The bulk of the palpitations had gone, at least the big ones. The dreadful cramps disappeared. The nervousness became less.

Something was very wrong. As I have already stated I had had a blood test for thyroid function and it was returned in the "normal range". I was determined to find why the result was "normal" when I obviously wasn't in normal health. After all, I am now being treated for hypothyroidism and I am very very well.

After eleven months of treatment, I could hardly believe how I felt. For the first few months I used to pinch myself just to make sure I was awake.

Sometimes, when we have been shopping and are making our way back to the car I do a hop, skip and jump just for the thrill of it. Norman prayed for my health and now I have my health.

CHAPTER FOUR

MEMORY LANE

I would like to go back a little further than twenty three years. I suffered from polio when I was eleven-and-a-half years old and wore a calliper on my left leg for twelve months. I couldn't attend school but was given work to do at home. Upon returning to school, I remember the gym mistress shouting at me because I couldn't climb up the ropes in the gymnasium. My arms were just not strong enough. I had a lot of trouble concentrating on lessons and my energy level had dropped drastically after polio. I never, ever, had the same stamina again, until now.

Looking back, my quality of life has been poor for most of it. There were times when I had periods of feeling better but every time a shock to the system was experienced, my health declined. It could be anything from, an operation, accident, birth, bereavement, or undue stress over a long period. Throughout my life, I have been susceptible to infections with numerous bouts of tonsillitis, cystitis, bronchitis, gum abscesses, pleurisy and womb infections. I was hospitalised three times with kidney infections.

Six of the misdiagnoses are clues in themselves.

1	Coeliac disease	malabsorption – food material not absorbed properly by the small intestine.
2	Epilepsy	
3	Depression	due to long term illness
4	Polymyalgia Rheumatica	muscular disorder
5	M.E.	entero virus, found in blood sample (I had polio aged 11 years).
6	Myasthenia gravis	serious weakness of certain muscles

Affected areas:

- Nervous system
- Brain
- Heart
- Skin
- Muscles
- Voice Box
- Hair
- Ears
- Nails

The thyroid gland is responsible for the energy transformation in every single cell in the body. Is it any wonder that there is such a diversity of signs and symptoms? Despite the fact that I was showing excessive signs and symptoms, my condition was not picked up on.

I was determined to research this until I found the answer. Through my investigations, I realised that there were a lot of sufferers out there whose diagnosis for hypothyroidism had been missed. I called these, "missed cases".

I was given a book to read, written by Dr. Broda Barnes of America. He spent forty years treating missed cases of hypothyroidism and his book was fascinating. He kept stating that the blood tests for thyroid function were unreliable and this information pointed me in the right direction, for my first serious research into hypothyroidism.

The library was my next port of call, where I pored over books on the thyroid gland, then concentrated on the understanding of the blood tests for thyroid function.

The thyroid gland is part of the endocrine system which comprises:

Pituitary, Thyroid, Pancreas, Adrenals and Gonads (testes in the male and ovaries in the female).

All these glands are interrelated and work together.

Everything was beginning to make so much sense. The endocrine system is made up of five main parts and three of mine were failing. No wonder I was in poor shape!

Thyroid disease is insidious. It creeps up on you and can take many many years for it to become full-blown. Although the misdiagnoses were over a period of twenty three years, I am sure that I was affected from the age of twelve after polio, bringing the total number of years to forty-three.

Because I had been ill for so long, my first thought was, will it work? Then will it last? When the first day of well-being hits you, you cannot quite believe it. Is it a trick of nature or is it psychological? How many times had I heard that over the years? As time passed, there was a little stirring in my brain that said it was going to last.

I well remember, when I had a few consecutive days of feeling good, how I launched myself into a spring-cleaning session at home, something that had been denied me for a long time. What a mistake! The next day I was back to square one. Pacing myself was hard, because I was so excited about feeling better.

I love to use my brain now, and to be able to think clearly for the first time in so many years is wonderful. I used to get so muddled and confused and felt ashamed and then tried to hide my embarrassment.

I have drawn a graph representing my sliding health scale which appears on the following page...

Diana's Approximate Sliding Health Scale

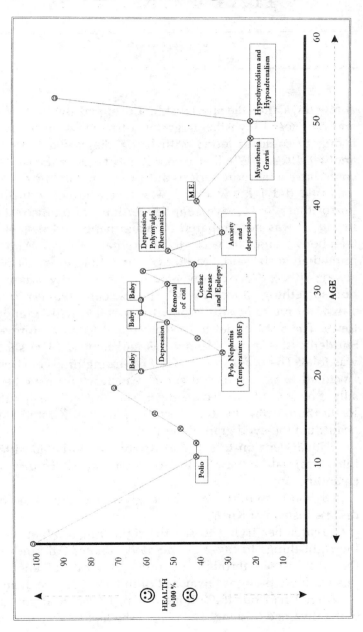

CHAPTER FIVE

KIRSTY

A few days after the specialist had dropped the bombshell and diagnosed myasthenia gravis, I had great difficulty in trying to come to terms with being diagnosed with yet another disease. Whether or not it was because the disease could have a far more serious outcome, I do not know.

Little did I know that I was to encounter a further horror that would leave a far deeper imprint on the rest of my life. I was not prepared for what happened next. The telephone rang. It was my daughter, Tanya. Almost immediately she said, "Mum are you sitting down?" I was always sitting down and wanted to joke with my daughter but something stopped me. The obscure request from Tanya for me to be sitting down was veiled with ominous tones. The silence that followed seemed to go on forever. Suddenly she spoke, "Kirsty has leukaemia." The shock was total! The brain works very fast during times of stress, I wanted to say, "Are you sure?" which would have been silly. She would not have rung if she had not been sure. Realisation came in and I said, "No, not Kirsty." My beautiful blue-eyed granddaughter.

Tanya went on to say that Kirsty was to be admitted into hospital immediately to start on a course of chemotherapy.

Oh God, couldn't you have given me this dreadful disease instead of Kirsty!

I remember trying to say the right things. What were the right things to say, does anybody know? All kinds of thoughts passed through my mind at a rate of knots. I pushed these thoughts away as I didn't want to face them.

After I had put the 'phone down, I tried to digest all that Tanya had told me. The reason she had taken Kirsty to the G.P. in the first instance was because she kept climbing up onto the couch and falling asleep. I must tell you that Kirsty was only fifteen months old when she was diagnosed. My daughter did not worry too much for the first few days, thinking that Kirsty had a virus. Then she noticed a series of small raspberry coloured bruises on her legs. The bruises concerned her.

At that time, there had been a great hullaballoo about mothers beating their children. Tanya knew that she had to take Kirsty to the doctor's, although at the back of her mind she wondered what the G.P. would say about the bruises. I cannot imagine how she felt being told that her daughter had leukaemia. I know what I was feeling for her and my son-in-law, Ian and I prayed to God for the courage they would need for the coming months. For my granddaughter, Kirsty, I prayed for strength for her little body.

The G.P.'s advice to Tanya and Ian was that Kirsty would have to be admitted into hospital straight away if she was to have any chance of survival.

At this point, I must tell you that Kirsty had a twin brother, Thomas. We will never know the heartache that Tom suffered during those long separations because of the time Kirsty spent in hospital. Unless we are a twin, I suppose we never will understand.

We all watched Kirsty change from a bright blue-eyed angel into a pale dark-eyed little girl who was so poorly. The medication played havoc with her little body. She received high doses of steroids and chemotherapy. Doctors came and went, medication was given many times in the day. Lots of trips to the theatre for the medical staff to take samples of spinal fluid and she took it all in her stride. She was an inspiration to us all!

She was quite beautifully bossy with the doctors sometimes and they loved it. She would tell them what they had forgotten.

Then she came home and started to pick up and we felt that the medication was working. She started to be able to play again which was wonderful to observe. By this time, I had to use a buggy to get around in and I would chase Kirsty and Tom in the park. Kirsty was in good health for seven months. Then she became unwell again and was taken into hospital and this time she was to be given more treatment. The frustrations and confusions that Kirsty must have gone through at that time must have been awful, besides feeling unwell in her body. I am sure that she must have wondered, in her own little way, what was going on.

The months went by and she was now aged two years. It was decided that they would try a bone marrow transplant. Now the question was who was to be the donor? Tom of course, was the obvious choice but when tests were carried out it was Kirsty's elder brother, Ben, aged six, who would be the most compatible. Ben was asked would he give some of his bone marrow to Kirsty. He said, of course he would and we all knew he would do anything for his beloved little sister.

The day before Kirsty was to have the bone marrow transplant she was allowed out for the day. Norman and I took Tanya and Kirsty to Knowsley Safari Park. She had come through so many bouts of being too ill to move, never mind a day out but the day we took her to the Safari Park she was full of beans. She enjoyed every moment of her day. The bouncy castle, the big car ride, the sea-lions and the other animals

It was her last day of fun.

Kirsty had the transplant and for a while she was all right but then she started to be unwell again. At three years and four months, she died in her sleep.

You may wonder why I am relating this story to you. The reason is because I do not know how Kirsty's little body coped with all the medication, the steroids, chemotherapy, radiotherapy and then the bone marrow transplant.

Shock can be a major cause of thyroid dysfunction, whether it be due to an operation, high doses of medication, accident, bereavement, undue stress, etc. Sometimes, the thyroid can right itself but really in Kirsty's case the thyroid would have had no time to right itself.

Maybe the medical profession ought to look at the endocrine system more closely when patients are subjected to this type of therapy.

Each illness I was diagnosed with and the subsequent medication I was put on, sent me further down the road of ill-health but for me that was over a period of twenty-three years, for Kirsty it was two years.

I, personally, would like to see more research done in this field. When patients are on this type of therapy, check the thyroid gland, pituitary, hypothalamus and the adrenal glands. It is possible that the thyroid gland is exhausted and needs a boost. It may indeed help them to cope with the therapy. I witnessed my little granddaughter go through the horrors of this treatment and feel that it must have affected other parts of the body, i.e., the thyroid.

I know, Lord, that there is a reason for everything that happens on this earth but accepting Kirsty's death was very very hard.

To brave little Kirsty,

I love you.

CHAPTER SIX

OBSERVATIONS

NORMAN:

There is absolutely no doubt in my mind that the diagnosis of hypothyroidism saved Diana's life.

It sounds very melodramatic to say, "I thought she was dying," but that was the thought going through my mind in May/June 1994.

I don't want this to sound like a eulogy of my wife but I love her for so many things. She always tries very very hard to attain a quality of life for herself and those around her, no matter how she feels in herself. We are very close and I can argue that I know her very well but at times I had not realised how ill she had felt and what supreme physical effort she had had to make.

It you have a broken leg or arm, people are understanding and sympathetic towards your plight. Hypothyroidism is insidious because it can creep up on you over a long period of time and can be triggered in so many different ways. This condition can become very serious and life-threatening.

When I first met Diana the medical professional had diagnosed coaliac disease. For several years, she had to select foodstuffs very carefully to avoid anything that contained wheat flour. Have you got any idea how often wheat flour is added to commodities? When we first got together I found that shopping for groceries took ages – we had to read every label on products to ascertain the contents. Items I took for granted were restricted from her. This was my first experience of her reduced quality of life.

She used to suffer a lot of shooting head pains, so sharp that they made her cry out and stabbing pains in hands, arms and legs; "gremlins" she called them. The doctor thought they might be due to spondylitis at the top of the

34

spine and the resulting pressure on the nerves. She still has spondylitis but it rarely troubles her in this way now.

She used to look after the house beautifully, everything was cleaned, dusted and polished. I had no idea of the physical duress this put her under – it was her way of "fighting" the lack of energy. I was out at work all day not realising that a small cleaning job was taking her all day to accomplish – she did not admit to this until some years later.

Eventually, I noticed that she was having trouble climbing the stairs, having literally to haul herself up hanging on to the banister. My children had moved away and we no longer needed a four-bedroomed house, so we bought a bungalow.

For a while, she seemed to cope much better but she was starting to drop off to sleep wherever she sat. We would be chatting, seated in the lounge, and I could be responding to a point she had made, or question, and after a couple of sentences I looked across to find her fast asleep. She started to take naps in the middle of the morning/afternoon/evening but they were not naps as you or I know them. She would go into a deep sleep for 20 to 30 minutes, "the sleep of the dead," as one doctor put it. When she woke up her face had crease marks where it had been cupped into her hand and those marks persisted for hours not minutes.

She found that her energy level and muscle strength were dropping gradually and a doctor (not our own G.P.) thought that she might have M.E. (a blood test revealed an entero virus). We joined the M.E. Association. I say we joined because we are "partners for life" and I felt it imperative to learn as much about the illness as possible. We went to an M.E. Association Meeting. I found the venue very strange as it was held on the first floor of a Community Hall – Di could barely climb the steps, even with my assistance. We sat at the back of the hall and listened to the speaker with interest and observed the other M.E. sufferers around us. That night, we both reached the conclusion that she was *not* suffering from M.E. I told Di that nobody I saw in that hall was as bad as her. Nobody moved as slowly, or with so much obvious difficulty and distress.

There was no medication to assist M.E. sufferers at that time, in fact, it had not been recognised by the Department of Health as a certified illness.

Di continued to deteriorate very gradually until she reached a point where our G.P. referred her to a specialist (consultant physician) at the local Nuffield Hospital. He examined her and gave her a tensilon test and diagnosed myasthenia gravis. This was good news and bad news. Good news because at last we thought we knew what the problem was; bad news because mysthenia gravis is a serious muscle disease which cannot be cured (although it can be controlled) and is sometimes terminal. On medication, Di definitely improved but that in part was due to the high dose of steroids. The high dose of steroids caused her to put on weight and extra weight put extra stress on the already weak muscles!

The improvement was relatively short-lived. After two-and-a-half years, Di confided in me that the medication was "poisoning her system" as she was feeling so unwell and she asked her G.P. for help in weaning her off it.

During this period, I had bought her an electric scooter-chair which gave her life a new dimension – now she could go out and about in my absence during the day and was not forcibly "tied" to the home.

She mastered the driving technique in no time at all and I was as excited about it as she was – it was wonderful to see her pleasure. Now we could go out for walks – me on my feet and she in her buggy, something we had not been able to do for a few years.

Our G.P. supported her application for registration as a disabled person and this improved her quality of life enormously. We were able to park near to shops so that she could "take charge" of some shopping expeditions.

Previously, when using public car parks, she had barely been able to walk to the shops.

Other problems presented themselves. She began to lose control of her bowel muscles and on one occasion, when walking back to the car from the shops, she alerted me to her desperate need to go to the toilet. I suggested we returned to the larger stores to find a toilet but Di (a very fastidious lady) wanted to go home. We reached the car and as I drove off she burst into tears saying, "I'm so sorry, I'm so sorry!" She was dreadfully upset because she had been unable to control her bowel motion – not upset for her own sake but for mine because she thought the smell and the mess would revolt me. When you truly love someone you only feel for their hurt.

I have said that Diana relied wholly on me for transport, but that in itself became a problem. As soon as we had set off on a journey (perhaps to the local shops) she fell asleep and on a longer journey, of one or two hours, she slept the whole time. She became very nervous in the car, which was totally contradictory to her attitude when we first got together – she rather liked speed. I was used to travelling the motorway only in the fast lane but now Di insisted that I drove only on the inside or the centre lane – she was frightened by the proximity of the central reservation barrier. I think I found this very hard to come to terms with.

In 1991, Di could no longer continue doing the housework as it became too much of a struggle. Tearfully, she told me she would have to have some help but typically said she would pay whatever it cost to employ someone (from her meagre income of Permanent Health Insurance). Only she will ever know what a fight she had within herself to come to this decision.

In January, 1993, I was made redundant which coincided with the Permanent Health Insurers deciding that Diana was fit for work and refusing to make any more payments. (Be warned, readers of this book, if you too have similar insurance cover.)

We decided to go abroad for the winter of 93/94. I had not been able to find work and was not looking forward to the winter. We felt that the warm sunshine would do us both good. We let out our bungalow, sold our car and bought a motor home and set off for three months in Portugal and three months in Spain. It was not a raging success. Firstly, we had a lot of miles to cover and Di was by now a very nervous traveller. Secondly, she went to sleep a lot, as I have explained but I needed her to navigate for me (neither of us had driven through France, Spain, or Portugal before). Thirdly, her general physical condition worsened. She became, in my opinion, irritable and irrational. She also developed "new" physical problems, suffering from severe palpitations, sensitivity to cold and a "forgetfulness" (she left things in shops, e.g. sunglasses, her handbag, etc.) I had to follow her round to collect these items and generally look after her interests which she found annoying and which I did not want to do because I felt I was crowding her. It was a stressful period.

We returned home on 1st April, 1994. Only then did I realise what efforts Diana had made in the preceding six months to just simply exist. It was almost as though upon reaching the safety and security of her own home she was able to let go but which resulted in her strength, both physical and mental, declining quite rapidly. She could no longer drive her electric buggy because she did not have the strength to pull in the lever to operate "drive". She rarely slept through a night and suffered very severe cramps in her arms and legs and even around her back – cramps that persisted for half an hour and reduced her to tears frequently.

In the morning, she got herself washed and dressed and then had to sit in the lounge to rest. Sometimes I had to wash her hair for her and even bath her occasionally. To move from the lounge to the kitchen she had to steady herself with one hand on the wall.

There was a church almost opposite and she got great comfort from going there on a Sunday morning. Often, I had to walk across the road with her and a friend would bring her back at the end of the service.

Eventually, a friend passed her some papers to read, written by a doctor in Surrey, about hypothyroidism. Di thanked her friend but put the papers on one side for a while. She told me she did not want to know about another disease – after all the doctors had misdiagnosed her for years. She did read the papers at a later date and was stunned. It was as though she were reading about herself. She made an appointment to see the doctor six days hence. She said they were the longest six days of her life – she was full of hope and fear.

The doctor diagnosed hypothyroidism. "Can you do anything for me?" Diana asked. "Of course," the doctor replied. "I can make you better." After a few weeks of simple medication, in tablet form, she started to feel better. Gradually her strength returned and she started to lose weight.

Being the person she is, Di started to research the illness. Why was it so difficult to diagnose and why did the medical profession appear to know so little about it? And in typical style, she told me she was determined other people would not suffer as she had suffered. Her energy and determination and selflessness have amazed me. She has spent almost all of her meagre life savings on this project and had remarkable success in terms of helping other sufferers to make their doctors aware of the problems and the solution.

It is very sad that some people we thought were friends have had difficulty in coming to terms with the change in her. I think some people really did not think that there was much wrong with her. She is now so different she could not possibly have been really ill, could she?

Di used to be quite naïve and loved everyone but in recent months she has learnt some very hard lessons from people who have turned on her. We do not know why these people have changed their attitude but as Di says, "You have to get on with life and move on and if necessary leave these people behind." One lady has expressed jealousy of Di. Quite how she can be jealous of twenty three years of poor quality of life through illness I do not know! Or perhaps she is jealous of Di's new found vivacity and zest for life? I would have thought pleasure and perhaps understanding and encouragement would have been more appropriate!

Before Diana and I got together, we used to speak regularly on the telephone (we lived about 55miles apart) I fell in love with her voice, which I found very pleasant, soft, warm and musical. About three or four years ago, I remember commenting to her that on the phone she had begun to sound like an old lady. We have found that hypothyroid sufferers do tend to have voice "peculiarities".

For some years, Di was unable to sing at all, despite having performed on stage earlier in her life in amateur musicals. Now her voice is very clear once more, her breathing much improved and she loves to sing in church. She has a very strong Christian faith (which helped her enormously through the worst times) and now sings for 'God'.

Her strength of character and determination have amazed me throughout. Her purposefulness in helping others is an example I can hardly hope to follow. Her helpline keeps her busy on the telephone for eight or nine hours a day and could be for much longer but I insisted she gave herself a break. Even now she will pick up the 'phone if she hears a thyroid sufferer leaving a message on the answerphone who sounds particularly distressed. Whether it is eight o'clock on a Saturday night or even eleven o'clock on a Sunday night – when she knows she will be spending up to an hour talking to the person, encouraging them, giving them support and explaining matters to them because of their lack of understanding, not only of what is happening to their minds and bodies but also because G.P.s generally do not have the time to counsel such sufferers in the way that they need – she will do it.

Now she has energy and forcefulness to arrange a meeting with the Department of Health in London, gain support from the World Health Organisation and interest magazines in her story. Yet only months ago, when shopping in the supermarket, I would find her standing still, staring at the shelves in a trance, her mind apparently blank and seemingly unable to move. I had to move her on gently and I can tell you, I was frightened for her.

Di may be only 5′ 3″ tall (I call her "Dinkie") but today she is a giant to me.

MARGARET:

"Would you like to come over and have a cup of coffee?" invited Di within half an hour of our first meeting some seven years ago. As we chatted, walking very slowly from the church to the bungalow, where she lived, I was not then aware that walking slowly was necessary for Di, who was so ill.

She had been diagnosed with myasthenia gravis and I noticed, over the months that followed, how much more pain she was in and how her life became limited to the home.

Di had always taken an interest in her appearance and with her dark naturally curly hair and love of vibrant colours together with make-up (she is an artist) she never looked really ill when she went out.

My visits had to be kept short, maybe an hour, because Di used to become exhausted quickly. We used to laugh a lot and that not only hurt her head but it was very tiring for her. I watched her trying to get into a comfortable position on the settee, supporting her head because of the pain in her neck and spine. She was so pale and there were dark shadows under her eyes and her mobility was slowing down more and more as her condition worsened.

I didn't know then that Di had a beautiful singing voice. The sad part about it was that she was so breathless

41

all the time so that at church she was only able to sing the odd part of a line, it was all she could cope with. At times, she had to remain seated throughout the service shifting position and nearly always supporting her head with her hand. How I felt for her.

Soon she needed to lean on an obliging arm to go the shortest distance because her knees and ankles gave way and her wrists hurt.

I have always admired Di's courage because she made light of the nightmarish situation that had gone on for so many years.

I was frequently alarmed by the severity of her choking attacks and wondered if, one day, one would prove fatal.

My dear friend was crumbling before my eyes.

The next milestone was the buggy. Di made fun of this little machine and loved it when I couldn't keep up with her. Privately, I thought, in another six months' time, she would be in a wheel-chair.

By this time, Di was very heavy with a puffy face and had reached a stage when she could not use the buggy.

God is good. She was due to see a private doctor as a last resort. She had been mis-diagnosed so many times. This, she vowed, would be the last time she would see any doctor.

Norman and I were apprehensive because of the years of misdiagnoses. We didn't want her bubble burst again! Di was excited about her appointment and we prayed hard.

The rest you will have read and truly wonderful it is to see my friend today. She moves freely and so quickly. When I used to visit Di before the latest treatment, I would ring the doorbell when I arrived, then park my bicycle, locking it up, tidying my wind-blown hair and I would still have time to "write a letter or two" before she would painfully make her way to the door.

Hard to believe now! I don't have time to lock my wheels before she is there at the door smiling a greeting. She stands beside me in church and sings whole hymns with her beautiful voice. The weight is falling away and her eyes dance and sparkle with her new love of life.

My dear friend is not content to be improving, she is working hard to enlighten other patients and the medical profession.

I feel very privileged and humble to see my friend, more alert and enjoying life to the full.

CHAPTER SEVEN

SIGNS AND SYMPTOMS

When we are ill we have signs and symptoms that can tell the G.P.s what they need to know, and together with a clinical appraisal, they can relate them to a certain illness or disease.

- **Signs**: are outward evidence of disease, perceptible to an examining doctor. A sign is proof to a doctor, something that is visible to the naked eye or that he can hear or feel.

- **Symptoms**: There are many ways to describe symptoms. We are each of us individual and each has their own style of expression.

The signs and symptoms for an underactive thyroid are so diverse but that is because the thyroid is responsible for the energy transformation in every single cell in the body. Not only is it responsible for the physical well-being of the person but the mental well-being also.

The signs and symptoms listed below are in no particular order of preference or severity. I suffered these signs and symptoms and will try to explain my experience in as much detail as possible together with other people's experiences.

EXHAUSTION: There is a world of difference between somebody complaining of tiredness and somebody who is exhausted. When a person is truly exhausted they are without strength. Many times I confronted the doctors with the fact that I was tired all the time. Their stock reply was "We all feel like that from time to time." I have since

44

learned that the medical profession uses the expression "TATT" for people who are complaining that they are "tired all the time". If you become exhausted doing small jobs around the house (i.e. washing up the breakfast dishes and afterwards feel the need to sit down because standing alone exhausts you) that is the time to impress on your doctor that you are really exhausted.

In the waiting room at the doctor's surgery, I observed people and their energy. When they wanted a magazine from the table in the centre of the room they just got up walked over smartly, picked one up and returned to their seat. It doesn't sound much but for me that would have been expending energy that I needed when going in to see the doctor.

In the days when I used my motorised buggy there were times when I had no strength in my grip to pull the lever that propelled the buggy forward.

Waking up in the morning feeling as exhausted as when I went to bed was part of my life. Set out below are some expressions used by hypothyroid sufferers:

"Worn out", "no energy", "everything I do takes so much effort", "weary", "like walking through treacle", "done in", "fatigued", "tired all the time", "like wading through water", "My get up and go has gone".

GOITRE: A goitre is a swelling at the base of the neck. You can have a goitre and suffer no signs or symptoms at all. Or you can have a goitre with hypothyroidism (underactive thyroid) or hyperthyroidism (overactive thyroid).

LETHARGY: Some people do not reach the exhaustion stage but instead are in a state of lethargy and have no motivation.

DIZZINESS: Most of the symptoms that I suffered were distressing, some more than others. The dizziness that I experienced over the years was most distressing. I couldn't turn around without feeling dizzy and yet most doctors dismissed it. I couldn't dismiss it, I had to live with it. At night, many times I awoke feeling very dizzy and it could last for hours. My face lost colour and I felt very ill. Repeatedly, I was so frightened that I awoke my husband and I never liked doing that but I thought I might die and I wanted to be with him.

There are two presentations of an underactive thyroid.

1. The patient is overweight and puffy.
2. The patient is thin and looks worn out.

WEIGHT GAIN: Over the last ten years of my illness, I had put on a total of 3st in weight. At 12st 5lbs and for my height of 5'3" I certainly looked and was overweight. Nobody likes to be overweight and I challenge anyone who says that they do. Needless to say, I did not like it. I became depressed about my weight and no amount of dieting helped to reduce it. With some the weight can shoot up over a very short time, i.e. some thyroid sufferers have put on over one stone in a matter of weeks without there being any change in eating habits. Some contacts have been backwards and forwards to the doctors to be told that they must be "cheating on their diet".

Once on thyroid replacement therapy I lost 9lbs in weight without trying. This weight loss I called my "thyroid weight".

After six months on treatment I decided I was well enough to try a calorie controlled diet to lose some more weight. I made a conscious decision to wait that long before trying a diet because I had been ill for a very long time and I wanted to give my body a chance to recover. I did not want to incur any undue stress on my body and felt the need to give my body the chance to repair. The diet worked. From 11stone 10lbs, I went down to 10½ stone. I could lose a bit more if I wanted to but I am happy with that for the time being.

SWOLLEN ANKLES: My ankles and feet had been swollen for so long. I had gone up in shoe size from 4½ to 5½. If I had been on my feet all day maybe I could have understood but most of my day was spent lying prone because I was so exhausted. I am now back to a size 4½ shoe.

PUFFY FACE AND HANDS: I used to look at my face and think what a mess, it was so puffy and pale. The lids were so baggy my eyes were practically closing. I kept telling doctors my face didn't look right. It was no good. I don't think they understood. My hands were like fat splodges and the rings cut deep into my fingers. Now I have problems keeping the rings on my fingers. I really must take my rings to the jewellers for them to make them smaller!

THICK TONGUE: My tongue was literally too big for my mouth. Once I had cleaned my teeth in the mornings (that was an exhausting job) I opened my mouth and looked at my tongue (which was covered in a disgusting yellow and white fur) and down the side of my tongue there were teeth marks. It actually felt big. I had trouble getting my tongue round some words because of its size. I did not know that this was yet another sign of hypothyroidism. My tongue is now normal size.

DRY SKIN, COARSE SKIN! My skin, for many years, was so dry and flaky. My facial skin had the texture of sandpaper and my knees, elbows and heels had hard crusty patches on them. No matter how much moisturiser I used it was all to no avail. My feet were in a very poor state. There were great crevices of thick dry skin, that split and sometimes bled. The skin on my face is now so smooth. My skin is in much better condition all round, bearing in mind that I am now 55 years of age.

BRITTLE NAILS: Soft, forever flaking.

DRY HAIR: My hair was limp and fly away and very fine. I was blessed with naturally curly hair so most of the time it did not look too bad. My head hair had thinned. Some people lose a lot of head hair.

HAIR LOSS OVER PARTS OF THE BODY: I lost most of my pubic and underarm hair many years ago and once again put it down to my age, not realising that losing one's pubic and underarm hair is not a pre-requisite for getting older. Most of my body hair has returned.

THINNING EYEBROWS: This was yet another sign. If only I had known then what I know now. My eyebrows were very thin and the outer edge was non-existent. My eyebrows are now normal.

FEELING COLD: Feeling cold when everybody else is warm. Sometimes I felt sick with cold, so much so, that it made me cry. My hands and feet were always cold.

OVERHEATING: Sometimes my body actually overheated. This sounds contradictory but if we think of the thyroid gland as the thermostat of the body then it doesn't sound so improbable. A wonky thermostat can play up either way.

HEADACHES: Blinding headaches that went on and on. Sharp shooting pains inside my head. Strange sensations in my head like shivering inside. These shiverings came on in different parts of my body as well. My head felt as though it was going to explode many times. That was quite frightening. Try explaining that one to the doctor!

MIGRAINES: Migraines are the worst kind of headache with all the accompanying symptoms such as light sensitivity, flashes of colour and zig zags before the eyes, vomiting and just feeling nauseous. Having to lie down in a darkened room sometimes for days. This can also be part of a thyroid problem. I suffered from this many years earlier but not in the latter years of the illness.

ACHING LIMBS AND JOINTS, CRAMPS: I hurt all over; muscles, bones and joints. If anybody touched me, a little more than gently, it hurt. We had to move from a house to a bungalow because I had great difficult in climbing stairs. Getting out of a chair had its problems as well. Cramps were another dreadful symptom. When they started it was agony. The cramps attacked my neck, back, hands and feet with real severity. I used to cry out, I was in so much pain.

LOWER BACK PAIN: An incessant pain that does not go away.

CARPAL TUNNEL SYNDROME: Bad pains at the wrists which makes the fingers tingle and become numb.

PALPITATIONS: Initially, they started out as just flutters. Towards the end of the illness they had become frightening episodes in my life. The palpitations would bang away inside my chest until I felt that my heart would burst. My heart was throbbing and trembling. At the end, they were coming every few minutes on some days. I thought that I was dying and so did my husband. He looked so drawn and worried and I couldn't relieve his mind because I felt so poorly. You may also experience ectopic heart beats (these are missed beats). It feels a bit like suddenly going down in a lift.

SHORTNESS OF BREATH: I suffered shortness of breath so much that I was diagnosed as asthmatic and had to take inhalers, the full prescribed dose of Ventolin, eight times a day and sometimes in between and the steroid inhaler Becotide four times a day. I now have one puff of ventolin every week or so. I used to wheeze for most of the day, now I don't wheeze at all.

DEAFNESS: Deafness seemed to have been with me for a long time but conversely there was something far more disturbing that was happening. I had over-sensitivity with my hearing. I picked up sounds that most people could not. I could hear everything that was going on in my husband's mouth when he chewed his food. Noises sometimes actually hurt my ears. I heard shooshing noises, ringing and high pitched whistling. I often accused my husband of mumbling. He complained that the T.V. was too loud. My hearing is now normal and the sensitivity has gone.

PALLOR: I just don't remember when I last had a rosy complexion. It must have been when I was at school. My facial colouring was pale and yellowy and there were little blue/black areas on my lips. Each morning I put on my make-up. I was always determined to try to look good even if I didn't feel it. Now – wait for it – I AM NOW PINK-SKINNED! and the blue/black areas around my lips have completely disappeared.

CONSTIPATION: I have been constipated all my life! Sometimes I could go for days without emptying my bowels and then when I did empty them, it was little hard dry lumps. I became very distressed when trying to empty my bowels. Straining brought on dizziness and strange sensations in my head and over my body. Now I empty my bowels on a daily basis with no problems – consistency normal.

DIARRHOEA: Many suffer with diarrhoea only. Some suffer with diarrhoea and constipation. Some contacts with irritable bowel syndrome have said that the condition has cleared up since they have been on thyroid replacement therapy.

SWOLLEN STOMACH: I looked between seven to eight months pregnant and most of the time I was uncomfortable. I thought I was eating too much. I wasn't eating too much! I did a calorie check, 1,000 was not too much! I am happy to report that my stomach is reduced to a fairly normal size.

MENSTRUAL PROBLEMS: I had not seen a period for the last two years of the illness. Prior to that I lost huge clots and I experienced a lot of pain with them. Many sufferers have very heavy bleeding and clots. With some there is cessation – when periods stop altogether.

A healthy woman starts her periods at puberty. At the onset of her cycle, her thyroid hormone levels drop and when her period has ended her thyroid hormone level goes up. Hence the discomfort at period time. Pains, low backache, bloated stomach, constipation, heavy breasts, headaches and various other symptoms. With a low thyroid disorder the thyroid hormone level goes down and we find that these symptoms are with us most of the time.

SHAKY HANDS, SHAKY BODY, JUDDERING IN THE SPINE: Yes, I suffered these as well. The shaky hands were very much worse towards the end of the illness. I remember a few times, I shook all over my body. I called a nursing friend out. After about twenty minutes, it stopped as soon as it had begun. She didn't know what it was and to this day I still don't know. I only know that it has not occurred since I have been on thyroid replacement therapy. The 'juddering' spine (vibrations in the spinal column) was with me constantly. That has also disappeared.

PINS AND NEEDLES: I experienced pins and needles in my hands, arms, legs and in my head.

NUMBNESS: Numbness could strike at any time in the hands, arms, legs, the base of the spine and the back of my head. Many mornings I awoke only to find that I had "lost an arm". This initially frightened me. I had to use the other arm to locate the lost one. When I found it, it was dead. I moved it up and down with the good arm until the circulation came back, which took some considerable time and was most uncomfortable. I must tell you that I was not lying on that arm when I woke up.

DECREASED SWEATING: I had noticed for the two years before diagnosis that I did not perspire as much. Some experience heavy sweating.

HOARSE VOICE: My voice became that of an old woman, according to my husband. I remember trying to impress on one specialist that the voice that was talking to him WAS NOT MINE. I think he thought that I had lost all my marbles. I went on to tell him that over the years my voice had changed considerably. He wasn't impressed. In fact, he dismissed it. Was this yet more evidence that I was getting older? I was never afraid of getting older but this was ridiculous. It wasn't happening to other people of my age. I began to accept it as my lot! My voice now, incredible to me, is back to what it once was.

DRY MOUTH, SORE THROAT: Continual. I also had the feeling that something was stuck in my throat – like a fishbone.

SWALLOWING DIFFICULTIES: I felt, sometimes, that there was a lump in my throat. The muscles in the back of my tongue were quite weak and I suffered choking fits over food and drink and sometimes, just on my saliva. These were frightening episodes in my life as I wondered which day would be my last.

SLOW SPEECH: My speech was so slow and deliberate. Sometimes getting my tongue around the words was so difficult. I could not speak any faster if I tried. Many times the brain would tell me one word and my mouth would say another, I found it very embarrassing. Often I forgot what I was talking about mid-sentence. I stumbled over words, said words back to front, I slurred my words and became tongue-tied on many occasions. I very often transposed letters in sentences so that instead of "I'll peel the carrots," it came out, "I'll ceel the parrots." The family and I had many a laugh at my new language. I have no difficulty now. In fact, I am most articulate.

SLOW THINKING: My thinking processes had slowed down so much and I had to think long and hard before saying anything. The moment was gone sometimes before I could think what to say.

LOSS OF APPETITE: I felt nauseous sometimes so did not feel like eating.

HIGH BLOOD PRESSURE: I did not suffer with high blood pressure, many do.

ALLERGIES: Skin allergies, skin sensitivities, burning of the face, so much so that you feel you are on fire. This is totally different to flushing due to the menopause. One lady told me that she had to keep putting cream on every hour because her face was becoming wizened with the burning. She called them "flare-ups". Alcohol made this condition worse for myself.

SENSITIVE TO THE SUN: I never used to be so sensitive. I found it made me feel ill to be in the sun. I have no problems with the sun now.

LOSS OF BALANCE: I lost balance many times when walking and veered off my course, to the left.

PAINS OVER HEART AND CRUSHING FEELINGS IN THE CHEST: I suffered a squeezing in the chest and thought I was having a heart attack. These feelings can be very distressing.

POOR MEMORY AND CONCENTRATION: When I was at school, I had problems concentrating. I always have had, throughout my life, especially the last twenty years or more. My concentration is now excellent. For the last four years, I have thrown myself in researching the problem of missed cases of hypothyroidism and diagnosed treated cases of hypothyroidism who are still not well and I have had no problem whatsoever with concentration. My memory was not good at all. Memory now excellent.

MORBID THOUGHTS: Sometimes, when Norman had left for work I visualised a fatal accident and would then live through the aftermath of funeral arrangements and how I would cope long term. Thoughts that maybe I had cancer or leukaemia. Many times thoughts of suicide were very strong.

SLEEPLESSNESS: The kitchen was my first stop most nights, when I couldn't sleep. A cup of tea was the first thing I thought of. Typically English, I know. I was as quiet as I could be in case I awoke my husband. I wandered round the house at a snail's pace and when I was tired, I sat down and read for a while. That did not last long because it hurt my eyes. After two or three hours, I crawled back into bed, exhausted and slept the sleep of the dead and then woke up even more exhausted. When I did sleep, I sometimes snored.

NIGHTMARES: Good dreams, bad dreams, strange dreams.

VISUAL DISTURBANCES: My eyes ached. When I looked from one side to another they ached. I had dry eyes that felt very gritty. I was light-sensitive. Some people's eyes are very sore. My eyelids were swollen and puffy. I suffered from blurred vision for many years, also poor focusing. I do not now suffer with any of these eye complaints.

ANGER AND IRRITABILITY: I was irritable and irrational, with constant mood swings. I know now that this was part of the illness.

NERVOUS AND JUMPY: Yes, I was in a very nervous state for a long time. Towards the end of the illness, I jumped at the slightest thing that moved. When drifting off to sleep at night, many times my body often jumped off the bed and my heart pounded in my chest and I became very distressed. This happened so many times, that I became afraid to go to bed.

PANIC ATTACKS: This was a very distressing part of the illness. It could happen day or night, at any time. There was no pattern to it. Suddenly things would not feel quite right and then I felt an agitation inside and without further ado, my heart raced away. It felt as though it were coming out of my chest. I became frightened of my own body and used to run into another room to try and get away from the feeling, all to no avail. This, of course, was silly because I could not run away from it. To say the least, it terrified me. What was happening to me? On occasions it took over two hours before it settled down. If anyone has experienced this, then they know what I'm talking about. The attacks were put down to anxiety. I do not suffer these attacks at all now. After six months of treatment, they completely subsided.

ANXIETY: I was anxious most of the time. It seemed to come from deep down inside me. The last ten years of the illness were the worst. Tasks that once would not have worried me became such a big issue that I became a "jibbering wreck". Again, this was put down to stress.

HALLUCINATIONS: I saw spiders coming out of the walls and they were BIG and REAL. Sometimes, when I looked at a person, their head would take on the appearance of someone else. This happened only in the last nine months of the illness. It was the most horrifying experience to go through.

VOICES IN THE HEAD: Yes, I heard voices, voices that told me to do things, such as "Mess the house up," "Put marks on the dining-room table," and many more things, too dreadful to state in this book. I became frightened of my own body. Many times, thoughts of suicide came into mind.

GUILT: I felt so guilty about being so unwell and at one time, doubted my own perceptible abilities. I found myself on the defensive most of the time and not liking myself at all. My self-esteem was at its lowest ebb.

SUSPICIOUS OF PEOPLE'S MOTIVES: Why were they doing things for me? Was there an alternative motive?

PERSECUTION COMPLEX: I felt people were talking about me behind my back. I not only felt it, I was convinced.

CRY OR GET UPSET EASILY: I cried at the slightest thing. In fact, I was very emotional and that doesn't help when you attend the G.P.'s surgery because he immediately thinks you are a neurotic, overweight woman who is depressed. There is nothing you can do about it because that is what is happening to you.

CONFIDENCE: I had lost confidence for many years. It took a long time for it to return. Taking journeys on my own was, at first, an absolute nightmare. It took many months and determination to overcome feelings of panic. If you are not feeling very confident, then persevere, it will get better.

CLAUSTROPHOBIA: I was afraid of being in confined spaces. I hated going to the toilet! I couldn't wait to get out. The shower cubicle was a no-go area for me because I had to be in there too long. I had a bath instead and even then I was in and out. I used to laugh at myself occasionally when I wasn't feeling too frightened. I have since stood in the smallest room of the house and in the bathroom for quite a while and revelled in the fact that I am no longer afraid.

AGORAPHOBIA: I felt very afraid to be in wide open spaces.

MOOD SWINGS: Mood swings were a part of my life for a long while. Sometimes I was totally unreasonable. Since becoming well, on thyroid replacement therapy, I have realised that before I was well my reasoning, my attitude towards people and what I thought was people's attitude towards me, was badly affected. Occasionally, I became very angry, sometimes for very little reason.

DEPRESSION: I was depressed. I defy anyone not to be depressed with all of these symptoms.

LIBIDO: Non-existent. This could, of course, be due to exhaustion. For a long time, after I became well, I had a mental block and it was only after many discussions with my husband that things improved.

HEAVY EYELIDS: My eyelids felt so heavy most of the time that I just wanted to close them and go to sleep. My eyes are now open wide and bigger than I remember them.

GENERAL PROBLEMS:

I lost my balance every time I walked a few paces. I was always bumping into things.

The palms of my hands were red hot and itchy.

I could not tolerate alcohol any more, it made me feel ill.

My head felt too heavy and many a time I had to hold it up with my hands. My limbs also felt heavy.

For those with flushed colouring, did you know that there is such a condition called **florid hypothyroidism**?

I found it very difficult to open tins. If I tried to put pressure on to the tin opener my fingers contorted into something quite grotesque.

One lady who contacted me said that she thought she had had a stroke because of the numbness.

According to my dentist I clenched my teeth. He said I was wearing away the enamel. I remember doing this sometimes in the day, he said I probably did it in my sleep as well.

I lived with fear most of the time because of what was happening to my body. I couldn't get away from it. I was frightened of my own body and locked into it and I couldn't get out. I now have a wonderful sense of freedom.

After waking up, I often found myself dribbling. This never happens now.

If too many people were talking at one time I became confused and couldn't make out the gist of what they were saying.

Crowds were a nightmare. I can now stand in a supermarket and revel in the people as they go about their business.

An outing in the car became a nightmare. At one time I loved speed, then I hated it. I thought that the verges or the barriers were coming straight at me. I now love speed.

I needed my personal space very much and sometimes just wanted to be on my own. I felt very guilty about how ill I was and if I was on my own I didn't have to lie about the way I felt. You feel a bit like a record that is played over and over again. I suffered very low self-esteem and tended to think that this was my lot. I couldn't fight any more.

The hallucinations, voices in the head and the paranoia I kept to myself. There was a reason for this. I had shared a lot with doctors and specialists over the years and had been misdiagnosed six times with serious diseases and treated for them. I thought that if I shared these symptoms they would probably lock me up. So I kept them to myself. I went through agonies in doing so.

Some lose their sense of humour.

My sense of smell was heightened.

If ever I had thoughts about what it was like to be an alien, then this was it.

I became an emotional "jibbering wreck". I couldn't stand to be touched by anyone. I was far less tolerant of people. I dissolved into tears at the drop of a hat or I simply wanted to hide away. I could not cope with any kind of stress.

I was very weak during the latter part of the illness and forced myself out of bed each morning because the thought of being bed-bound horrified me.

My whole view of life became very distorted.

In retrospect, I was totally frustrated with everything that was happening to me and the fact that I could no longer take part in real living. My quality of life was very poor.

I manifested most of the above signs and symptoms.

I needed to be understood by the medical professional not patronised. I was vulnerable at that time. Sometimes, we are treated very insensitively.

I felt so alone, nobody heard me – I mean the medical professional. Yes, they listened BUT THEY DID NOT HEAR. If any of you reading this book are suffering or have suffered you will understand. As a point of interest I itched everywhere on my body, so much so that it drove me to distraction. The whole body appears to be drying out: dry skin, dry hair, dry nails, dry eyes,, dry mouth, dry vagina. Certain secretions are more viscous in nature, for example nasal secretions.

Hypothyroidism is insidious. Signs and symptoms creep up on you so slowly that they become the norm. They are uncomfortable in the first few years and then they reach a stage when they are more than uncomfortable and you start your regular trips to the doctor. You end up going to see him more times than you would like but things keep happening to you. One week one set of symptoms is to the fore and in a few weeks' time, another set of symptoms is to the fore. It is not your fault it is happening. One important point – OVERACTIVE signs and symptoms overlap with UNDERACTIVE signs and symptoms, for example fast pulse, irritability, mood swings, etc.

After so many years, the doctor thinks that you are depressed. Of course you are depressed with everything that is happening to you but it is a reactive depression and not a clinical depression.

In a later chapter, I will try and help you to prepare yourself for your visit to the doctor's surgery.

This has been my story, a long one, sometimes difficult to write because of the distressing things that have happened to my body, both mentally and physically but the story has been necessary because it is everybody's story who thinks they may be suffering from a thyroid problem or who are diagnosed and treated and yet still not well.

Thank you, God, for my present health.

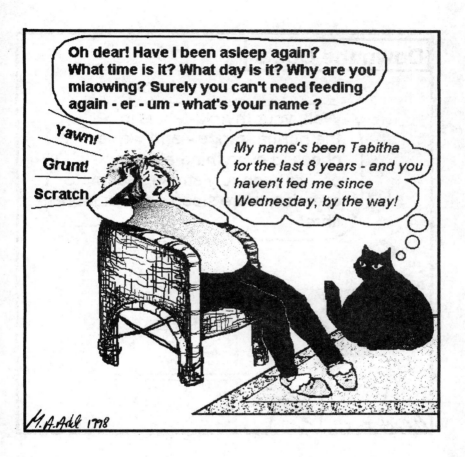

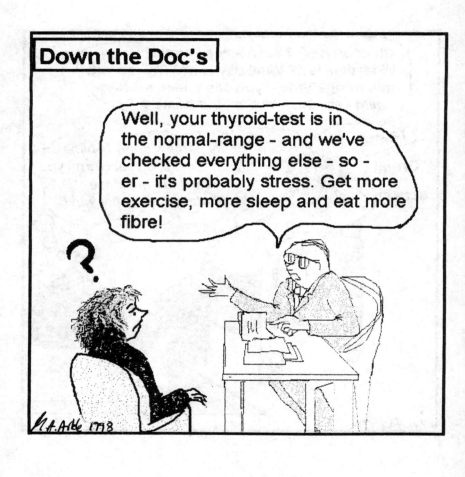

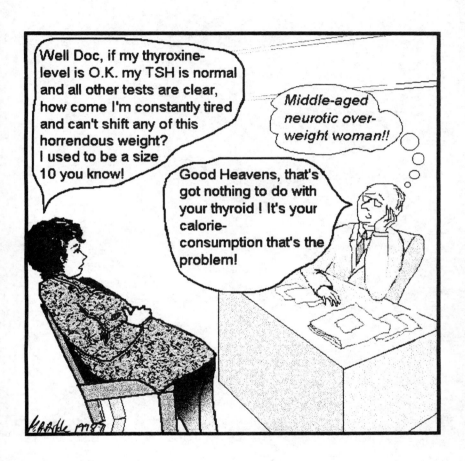

CHAPTER EIGHT

RESEARCH

Once I was feeling so much better and my concentration and thinking processes were much sharper, I knew that I had to find out why the illness from which I suffered had not been picked up before. Eighteen months prior to being correctly diagnosed, I had had a blood test for thyroid malfunction. The result was returned "normal range". Yet I had been ill for so many years.

I had read books and papers written by Dr. Broda Barnes of America. He had studied hypothyroidism for over forty years. After listening to tapes by Dr. Barnes, I was interested in what he had to say. He stated that we each had a biochemical identity and although the blood test can show how much hormone is in the blood, the blood test cannot tell us how much is necessary for the health of each patient, or indeed how much is usable. He also stated that there may be a conversion problem from the hormone T4 to T3. All this led me to believe that the blood tests can tell us much but that they are not specific enough.

I decided to go back to basics and find out how the tests for hypothyroidism were carried out.

BLOOD TESTS FOR THYROID FUNCTION

According to Sir Richard Bayliss, an eminent endocrinologist, the reference values for testing blood for thyroid function are "95% fiducial limits of so-called healthy people," which means, "an assumed fixed basis of comparison of so-called healthy people." This is very loose, but it is not the starting point that is the problem, it is the end interpretation. Doctors stick rigidly to the parameters set for the reference values. If there is flexibility with the starting point then there must be flexibility upon interpretation.

I was concerned about the "normal range" blood test results returned. Who is to say that one person's "normal range" is the same as another?

I decided to write to the World Health Organisation. Their reply was encouraging. Stated below are some of the comments they made.

26/7/94

"Dear Mrs Holmes,

"You rightly say that the "normal range" may not be an appropriate reference for decision making. Indeed this is why laboratory experts are recommending to abandon the term "normal range" and replace it with 'reference interval', while keeping in mind that the limit values for the 'reference interval' will depend on the selected population that was investigated for their establishment.

"Experts in laboratory diagnosis of thyroid disease do not stop to point out that in individual cases the levels of thyroid hormone may well be within the so-called "normal range" in patients with thyroid disease and the existing disease can only be diagnosed properly by investigating the spectrum of factors contributing to the regulation of thyroid metabolism.

"It should also be emphasised, that there are considerable differences in result measurements for technical reasons and this is particularly true in hormone measurement. No doubt that the clinician must be aware of all limitations when taking care of a patient on the basis of laboratory investigations only. Unfortunately, we often observe an unsatisfactory communication between laboratory and practitioners which may in some cases be the reason for misinterpretation of laboratory results."

That reply was more than I could have hoped for. I was spurred on to find out about and advise more people of the problem.

I wrote to Dr. Mike Wall, a Director of Public Health Medicine in South Staffordshire. We had a meeting and he encouraged me to continue with my research.

My next undertaking was to write to the Department of Health. I received another favourable reply asking me to meet with officials in London to discuss the areas of concern. A meeting was arranged.

I carried on with the research into the problem of missed cases of hypothyroidism. Then someone told me about Caroline Hulme, a lady who ran a helpline in Manchester. She had been counselling thyroid sufferers for ten years. I needed to find out why they needed counselling. I was diagnosed and felt very well and did not feel the need to be counselled. I rang her and introduced myself and told her what I had been doing regards missed cases of hypothyroidism. What she told me was amazing! She counselled diagnosed *treated* cases of hypothyroidism who were still not well!!

This was a truly wonderful find. There was a two-fold problem here. On the one hand missed cases of hypothyroidism and on the other treated cases of hypothyroidism who were not yet well. Something was radically wrong here and I was determined to find out what it was. I had a hunch but I needed proof.

I asked Caroline about the patients' medication, those who were diagnosed and treated. It appeared that once diagnosed as being hypothyroid treatment is commenced. A blood test is taken shortly afterwards and once the hormone level is within the "normal range" they are told they are euthyroid (normal) and they don't need any additional medication. The fact that the patient is still suffering dreadfully seems to be of no consequence. These patients fall into the same area on the 'reference range' as the missed cases of hypothyroidism. Now I had found that there were even more people suffering – diagnosed treated cases who are still not well.

I looked hard at the two-fold problem that I was faced with. Why had nobody picked it up? I wrote another paper before I met with the officials from the Department of Health and sent it down to them. I also asked Caroline if she would attend the meeting as she had a valuable contribution to make.

The meeting was held and the official in charge, Dr. Peter Bourdillon, stated that he would record in summary form the nature of our discussion and send us some references.

Set out below is part of the summary sent to me from Dr. Bourdillon.

4/4/95

"Dear Mrs Holmes,

"You and your colleagues described two types of patient with hypothyroidism and from the number of letters you have received both types seem commonplace. In the first type a person is diagnosed as having hypothyroidism, is treated with thyroxine and the thyroid function tests return to "normal range". The person is not given the opportunity to see if a further increase in the dose makes them feel better still or actually makes them feel worse because they become hyperthyroid. In the second type the person has the signs and symptoms of hypothyroidism and 'normal' thyroid function tests; the diagnosis of hypothyroidism is then dismissed and the person is labelled with a number of other diagnoses, most commonly depression.

"There is a problem relating to the intra-individual day-to-day variability in thyroid function tests. The "normal range" for T.S.H. for instance, is roughly, 0.5 to 5 mU per mL. A change of greater than 0.8 mU per mL in an individual's measurement, assuming no intercurrent illness, is a significant change. Consequently a person having a T.S.H. of 1.5 on one occasion and subsequently a T.S.H. of 3.5 had had a significant rise in his/her T.S.H., yet both are within the "normal range". I said that were a person lucky enough to have repeat measurements of thyroid function tests, most physicians would say, "we have now had two tests of your thyroid function and both of them show that your thyroid is working normally."

"I suggested that there are two ways of handling the issue of day-to-day variability in thyroid function tests; one is to stimulate research and the other is to make patients with

64

treated hypothyroidism aware that they may benefit from a further increase in their thyroxine therapy even if their thyroid function tests are within the "normal range".

More thinking had to be done: there were still parts of the puzzle that were missing. Then it came to me. When doctors interpret blood tests for thyroid function they have no base-line to work from. The patients never had a blood test for thyroid function when they were well. Secondly, how many doctors know how the reference values are made up for thyroid function tests?

I was to write another paper. Set out below is part of that paper:

THE PARAMETERS SET AGAINST THE REFERENCE VALUES FOR THYROID FUNCTION TESTS ARE OPEN TO MISINTERPRETATION

The reference values for thyroid function tests are made up of "95% fiducial limits of so-called healthy people', this is very loose. The laboratory experts have to start somewhere and it is certainly not the 'starting point' that is the problem, it is the end interpretation. If there is flexibility at the starting point then there must be flexibility upon interpretation. **This is not happening! There is too much rigidity upon interpretation!!**

Doctors are allowing the blood tests for thyroid function to become the determining factor in diagnosis, instead of relying on the patient's signs, symptoms, history, clinical appraisal and using the blood tests as a guide only. Pharmacologists say that diagnosis, when using blood tests, should be in probable terms.

The World Health Organisation say that laboratory experts are to abandon the term **'normal range'** from the reference values and replace it with **'reference interval'**. Perhaps the word normal has been the culprit, it is a nice safe word to have around, especially in today's society, who will sue at the drop of a hat. The World Health Organisation also say that there is not enough communication between the laboratories and practitioners.

Some people in the middle to lower range of the blood tests for thyroid function may need to be in the upper range of normal or they could show manifestations of hypothyroidism.

Some people in the upper range of normal need to be lower down the range or they could manifest symptoms of hyperthyroidism.

There is a self-help line for hypothyroid sufferers in Manchester and 80% of their calls are from **diagnosed treated cases of hypothyroidism who are not yet well.** Once their hormone levels are inside the 'normal range', they are told they are euthyroid. The fact that the are still suffering dreadfully seems to be of no consequence!!

We have a three-fold problem here, and all because the parameters set against the reference values for the blood testing of thyroid function are open to misinterpretation.

THREE-FOLD PROBLEM

1. Treated cases of hypothyroidism, who are still unwell, are told by their doctors, that once their hormone levels fall within the 'normal range' of the reference values they are euthyroid even with outstanding evidence to the contrary. The fact that the patient is still suffering and is continuing to have poor quality of life seems to be of no consequence.

2. The above problem with treated cases of hypothyroidism, substantiates the problem with missed cases of hypothyroidism. Their hormone levels never go outside the 'normal range' of the reference values and because they are inside the 'normal range' of the reference values, are classified as euthyroid. They are suffering the same as treated cases who are in the 'normal range' and equally, their quality of life is poor.

3. Cases of hyperthyroidism whose thyroid hormone result is at the upper end of 'normal' may need to be further down the range.

Many times G.P.s and Consultants say, "your thyroid function test is in the normal range." It may not be 'normal' for that person.

Let us take an FT4 range of 10 - 24. Some people at 10 are very healthy and the same through to 24.

In an FT4 range of say 10 - 24 one person with a result of 13 with many signs and symptoms of hypothyroidism may need to be at the upper limit of 'normal' and vice-versa another person with signs and symptoms of hyperthyroidism at 22 may need to be at the lower end of the range. How do doctors know where your normal range is, they never did a thyroid function test when you were well.

How many doctors know how the reference values are made up?

Pharmacologists say that only a handful of GP's would know how the reference values are made up.

If the GP's do not know how the reference values are made up, then **how do they know how to interpret the results?** If they knew how loosely the reference values were made up, they might not be so rigid with their interpretation of the results. **How can they hope to diagnose or even manage the patient's medication, if they do not understand the reference values in the first place?**

With the observations made in this paper, this pre-supposes 'a wide margin of error'.

Why are the parameters of the blood tests so religiously adhered to?

Euthyroid means normal thyroid hormone levels.

My next target was the Royal College of General Practitioners. The reply I received from Dr. Bill Reith, Honorary Secretary of Council, was more than I could have hoped for.

Part of that letter is set out below:

23/10/95

"Dear Mrs Holmes,

"You do indeed highlight a problem that we have with many tests in that the reference ranges, by definition, include only 95% of normal people with respect to thyroid function tests. However, this should be less important because it is a disease whereby it is crucial to treat the patient and not the blood test result.

"For patients who are diagnosed as hypothyroid, whose blood test returns to within the reference range but are still unwell, then it would be very reasonable to treat the patient with thyroxine. For those patients who appear to suffer from hypothyroidism but whose blood result is within the reference range, then the general practitioner appears to have two options.

"One is to try a small dose of thyroxine to see if the patient clinically improves, or, secondly, to refer the patient for specialist opinion. Whatever action the G.P. takes, if the patient remains unwell, it would not seem unreasonable for the patient to be referred, even if the G.P. considers that he has excluded hypothyroidism as a diagnosis.

"Provided both the advantages and the disadvantages are explained to patients so that they can make an informed decision together with their G.P. then it seems unlikely that either patient or their general practitioner would be disadvantaged.

"I will agreed with your suggestion that further research in this area would be helpful. It is also important for general practitioners to be mindful that a small percentage of normal patients will fall out with the reference range and similarly, there will be a few abnormal patients who will fall within them."

Let us look at the letters of response to my paper on parameters.

The World Health Organisation states that most professionals working in the laboratory are aware of the limits of the interpretation of laboratory results and particularly border-line cases.

Why hasn't this information been passed on the G.P.s and consultants.

They also state that the laboratory experts are going to abandon the term "normal range" and replace it with "reference interval".

World Health Highlights:
- Limitations of the interpretation of laboratory results.
- Inappropriate reference for decision making.
- Uncertainty.

Department of Health Highlights:
- Day to day variability in thyroid function tests.

- Patients not given the chance to see if any increase in their dose of thyroxine makes them feel better or actually makes them feel worse because they become hyperthyroid.

Royal College of General Practitioners Highlights:
- It is crucial that the doctor treats the patient and not the blood test result.
- Try a small dose of thyroxine to see if the patient clinically improves.
- Further research in this field would be helpful.

The above statements indicate that the blood test for thyroid function is questionable and therefore open to misinterpretation.

I was in receipt of all this information – now what did I do with it?

My mind was buzzing, and something started to formulate. I had been diagnosed with M.E. The signs and symptoms for M.E. are the same as hypothyroidism. Could it be that M.E. sufferers are in actual fact hypothyroid or maybe have a multiple endocrine problem? I threw myself into more research. Yes, I believe that a large majority of M.E. sufferers are indeed hypothyroid. I was to write another paper on M.E. and The Endocrine Connection.

M.E. AND THE ENDOCRINE CONNECTION

It would appear that there are two groups of M.E. sufferers.

- **GROUP ONE:** Viral infection. Patient contracts viral infection and thereafter suffers from many viruses and there is a gradual decline in health.
- **GROUP TWO:** Gradual decline in health over a long period.

In both groups, patients have a multiplicity of symptoms all seemingly unrelated. The majority have numerous tests including blood tests for hypothyroidism with the result being returned "normal levels".

Unfortunately, a great deal of reliance is being placed on the parameters set against the reference values for the blood tests of thyroid function and low adrenal reserve. Blood tests should be used as a guide only and not be the determining factor in diagnosis. Tests can tell how much thyroid hormone is in the blood but not how much is usable at cell level. Some people in the middle to lower range of the reference values may need to be in the upper range of normal.

If diagnoses are made in probable terms taking into account the patient's signs, symptoms and history together with a clinical appraisal, maybe there would not be the many missed cases of hypothyroidism and patients suffering from adrenal exhaustion that there are today.

M.E. manifests the same signs and symptoms as hypothyroidism. Hypothyroidism can be brought on because of many reasons: e.g. virus, shock, accident, operation, bereavement, birth, overdose on medication, undue stress over a long period of time, etc. All these reasons apply to M.E. as well.

Patients suffering with M.E. still remain an enigma to the medical profession. **There are missed cases of hypothyroidism.** Surely it is not unreasonable to suppose that a large number of M.E. patients could be suffering from an endocrine deficiency.

A further thought: Let us take GROUP ONE. Supposing a condition existed before the onset of a virus, i.e. **sub-clinical hypothyroidism.** Sometimes, when a patient with this condition contracts a virus, recovery is conspicuous by its absence and the patient's health declines.

THERE ARE CLUES THAT POINT TO AN ENDOCRINE CONNECTION IN M.E.

1. Dr. P.O. Behan, Glasgow, suggested that M.E. is a metabolic disorder, caused by persistent viral infection and associated with defective immunoregulation. There are three clues here, **metabolic disorder, persistent virus** and **defective immunoregulation.** These three clues relate to a **thyroid malfunction.**
2. Scientific verification: A unique metabolic derangement in energy production in the muscle cells shown by magnetic resonance. With an **endocrine malfunction** the **metabolism** is **disorganised and disturbed.**

70

3. Outbreaks of viral infection: Many people are prone to viral infections, most regain their health after a short period of time. There is a core group who do not and they begin to manifest symptoms of M.E. or an **endocrine malfunction.**

If all cases of M.E. were to be re-assessed, taking the patient's signs, symptoms, history and a clinical appraisal and using the blood test as an indicator only, perhaps many cases of hypothyroidism would be picked up.

I do not advocate that everyone with M.E. is suffering from a thyroid condition, what I am saying is that everyone with M.E. should have their thyroid function test checked with someone in the medical profession who is up to date with the interpretation of thyroid function tests.

Dr Skinner does not treat M.E. patients with thyroxine. If patients are presenting with a thyroid condition, then they are treated with the appropriate medication.

It is my great pleasure to relate to readers of this book, that many M.E. sufferers have been diagnosed with an underactive thyroid condition and under the direction of Dr. Gordon Skinner, they are now enjoying a good quality of life.

CHAPTER NINE

HELP-LINE

Through Caroline Hulme in Manchester, *She* magazine contacted me and asked if I would be prepared to relate my story for the September, 1995 issue. This could be what I was looking for. If my 'phone number was put at the end of the article I could start a help-line and dissipate all the information I had received to other sufferers.

The response to the article was simply amazing and as a result I received over 300 calls. I thought that I had prepared myself for the telephone calls as I had armed myself with a pad and a pen. I was certainly not prepared for the onslaught.

People were quite nervous to begin with and then as they gathered confidence everything came out in a rush and I could not write fast enough and then had problems deciphering my notes afterwards.

Each call was taking forty-five minutes to an hour. By the end of two weeks, I was totally exhausted after having received 160 calls. I realised that I had to cut down on my hours on the 'phone or I would be of no use to anyone. I had taken on board all the hurt, pain and frustration and loneliness of these people.

I had a hard time being objective about the 'phone calls, having previously been as ill as these people.

I decided that if this was going to work and if I was going to be of use, then I would have to change my approach.

I made out a comprehensive list of signs and symptoms onto an A4 sheet and photocopied it. As the calls came in, I highlighted their signs and symptoms and asked various questions such as height, weight, any previous illnesses or operations and so on. This gave me a better picture and I kept these as case notes. In doing this, I saved myself a lot of time in that, when the contact rang again, their previous history was on file.

I offered the contacts a 'pack' which contained my paper on parameters and copy reply letters from the Department of Health, the World Health Organisation and the Royal College of General Practitioners. These they took along to their doctor's surgery. Many doctors viewed the papers and correspondence objectively and acted upon the information and as a result, their patient's health improved either by starting them on thyroid replacement or by increasing their dose. Not everybody who rang through had a thyroid problem but approximately 85% of them did.

The calls I received were a mixture of both cases who had been missed out in diagnosis and diagnosed treated cases who were still not well.

MISSED CASES:

This group gave varied accounts based on the same theme. Many were to tell me of the years of suffering with little or no help from their G.P.s. A few of the G.P.s were compassionate and frustrated because they could not determine diagnosis for the patient. Their blood test results were in the "normal range".

There are many G.P.s and consultants who are a disgrace to their profession. They show neither compassion nor sensitivity to the patient's predicament. This, in turn, makes the patient feel uncomfortable upon entering the surgery. They already suffer from a lack of self-worth and confidence and can do without insensitivity on the part of the G.P. or consultant.

I had one lady who wrote to me saying she felt that "doctor" ought to spelt G.O.D. For those G.P.s or consultants who fall into this category it would be better if they treated us as human beings and realised that we are not without intelligence. If only they would talk to us. If we want to know the result of our blood tests, why not give it to us, instead of treating it as an affront? Under the Patient's Charter we *are* allowed to see our records.

I wish the medical profession would realise that they do not have the monopoly on intelligence. Anyway, why all the secrecy? After all it is our body! If a G.P. or consultant is at a loss for a diagnosis, then why don't they have the grace to admit it? We are not going to condemn them for it. The medical profession has no right to intimidate or belittle us; they are supposed to be giving a service. The patient may not have been to medical school but when reason and logic come into play they are a match for any physician.

The kindest way in which a doctor can put his point over is by being gentle, remembering that the patient is unwell. If only they would listen. We would like to take some responsibilities for own well-being and while the G.P.s are being so secretive about our records it is hampering our progress.

Thank you to those doctors who already do this, unfortunately you are in the minority.

DIAGNOSED TREATED CASES WHO ARE STILL NOT WELL:

These patients have their hopes raised and then dashed because once their hormone levels return to just inside the reference ranges they are classed as "normal" by both G.P. and consultant. "You do not need any additional medication, the blood test dictates you are on enough thyroxine." The patients thought that their troubles were over and that they would become well. In the majority of cases this hasn't happened and so the depression and anxiety rates are rising. Why don't they try asking the patient? More often than not the patient tries to tell the G.P. or consultant how he/she feels but the physician couldn't be less interested. Many times, these patients feel it's their lot and put up with it. This nation is full of brave souls.

74

When contacts ring me, I can hear the relief in their voices, although they have had a hard time coming to terms with the fact that I actually believe them.

95% of the ladies that ring me have been diagnosed depressive and have been put on to, or have been offered, antidepressants.

It had become apparent that the blood test is being diagnosed now instead of the patient. While the present system for blood testing thyroid function is used, many more will go undiagnosed or will be receiving insufficient treatment.

The medical world has become too technical and is not taking into account that it is the patient who is endowed with the sense of feeling and not the blood test.

At this juncture, I must say that there are patients who are on thyroid replacement therapy and they are very well and leading a normal life.

This book is directed mainly at women because it would appear it affects women on the whole. Men are affected with this condition but why a minority? Another area for research, I think!

The health editor from *Woman* magazine approached me and asked me whether I would like to feature in their January 1996 issue. The response from this magazine was even more amazing. In seven months, I received over 1,000 calls.

With the number of calls that I am receiving I believe that the problem out there of missed cases and diagnosed treated cases who are still not well is much bigger than is yet known.

All of these patients are desperate to be well. It would appear that the medical profession seem to think that people want to be ill. Very few people fall into this category. Some have spent thousands of pounds in trying to do just that very thing – get well. Many come away from the G.P.'s or consultant's feeling belittled, just plain stupid or that the doctor had just not listened to them. Many are in tears and are afraid to face the doctor again when he had told them there was nothing wrong with them. If the patient has the audacity to voice an opinion then they really are in trouble. Some patients have been struck off the G.P.'s register – this I find particularly appalling!

The best advice that I can give to the patient is to be persistent and moderately assertive. With the information given in this book you will become more aware of how things are done and what responsibility you are prepared to take for your own body. Take somebody into the G.P.'s surgery with you.

Through my research, I learnt that when patients are diagnosed with hypothyroidism they are given an exemption certificate which enables them to have free prescriptions for all medications. Does it have to be for all medication, why can't it just be for thyroxine?

G.P. Fund Holding practices are in danger of becoming patient selective, especially when long term medication is required by a patient on free prescriptions!

CHAPTER TEN

OTHER STORIES

NORMAN HOLMES – MY STORY

Di asked me to write my story because it is fairly typical of middle-aged men and may help a lot of people out there.

I have always been fairly active and determined and have enjoyed sport without being particularly good at anything.

The first major trauma in my life came when I joined a partnership in north Wales (I am a chartered surveyor) and within a few weeks found that the financial information that had been provided by my two partners, neither of whom were professionally qualified, was false. One was honest but very naïve, the other one was basically dishonest and very manipulative. The dishonest one went to prison (three years after I left the practice).

Not only did I disrupt my family, moving them from the Midlands to north Wales and back to the Midlands again, all in the space of eight months but I lost, what was to me, a lot of money and was interviewed by the Fraud Squad in connection with their investigations into my former partner.

I lost, for a while, security, which I need as an individual, money which I needed for security and was afraid that I might somehow be involved in matters that were outside my control and which could result in my losing my professional qualification (and therefore what security I had by then regained and my only means of earning a living). I think I was a little traumatised by these events and it certainly affected my relationship with my (first) wife.

I went through a second very bad patch in my life when my first marriage broke up and for a long time felt very depressed and disillusioned.

Then I got together with Diana and began to enjoy life again. The children left home one by one and Di and I moved into a place of our own and we were both really happy.

Then, during an annual medical, I was told that I was suffering from high blood pressure. I knew there was something wrong, without knowing what it was and I think I am typical of a lot of men in that I do not like to consult the doctor. I even argued against taking medication for the problem because I felt that I could control the problem myself but was persuaded to take a daily pill with the doctor's words, "I don't want to be reminding you of this conversation when I am attending you following your first stroke!"

My position at work became quite pressured, particularly when a new chief executive was appointed and I was getting home each evening feeling really tired, due to stress, I thought.

Prior to my high blood pressure being recognised I had a powerful sports motor-cycle (a Honda V.F.R. 750cc). Motor-cycling had always been my passion, right from the age of twelve and this bike was the realisation of my ambitions. I loved going out with two (also aged) pals who both had sports motor-bikes. But after a few months, I found I could not handle the machine. I wanted to ride quickly but found that I could not cope with it; I was no longer riding smoothly as my judgement of speed and distance was awry.

I also found that I was struggling with D.I.Y. jobs around the home. Even cutting the lawns with a motor-mower was tiring me out. I put it down to my age (I was fifty) and years of stress and current pressure. How many more 45-50 year olds out there recognise themselves from this? ARE YOU FEELING YOUR AGE?

In January 1993, aged 53 years, I was made redundant, having been with the organisation for sixteen years. And boy was that a shock to my system!

I worked hard at trying to find another job but found that a lot of things I did needed effort instead of being second nature. I used to drive to Birmingham about three times a week to an "Executive Job Shop" and found many times that I was anxious on the journey, rarely exceeding 65 m.p.h. I had been used to travelling up and down the country on motorways in big powerful cars – I used to think nothing of driving down to London for a nine o'clock site meeting and being back in the office in Wolverhampton at lunch-time.

My memory seemed to be failing me from time to time too and I was sometimes aware that I was slurring my speech a little. I was also given to irritability. It was all due to my age and stress I thought, nothing that I couldn't overcome in due course. I was also losing my hair.

Unknown to me, Di, despite her own extreme difficulties, was quite worried about me. She recognised my deterioration more than I did!

Whilst on a visit with Di to her private G.P. she asked me if I would let the doctor look at me? How could I refuse, I was there! My reflexes scored "2 out of 10" and the doctor thought that I had a hypothyroid condition, albeit fairly mild. So, I reluctantly started to take the medication (more tiny tablets) and within three months felt very much better. The start of the treatment coincided with starting part-time employment with my son, helping him with his commercial carpet cleaning business. The first time I was involved was in a small job, lasting about three hours and when we had finished and loaded the heavy machines into the van, I sat down and felt I was going to die. I could not cope but I would not tell my son. Not only did I need the income, but I needed to feel wanted and above all I could not admit my frailty.

A few months later (and by now well into the medication for my thyroid condition) we squeezed two jobs into one day and the team was working for seventeen and a half hours, stopping only for lunch and tea and a half hour journey down the motorway from one location to the next and I was less tired at the end than my twenty one year old colleague.

I now have a job as a surveyor again, working on an average of ten hours a day, working to tight deadlines, financial targets and in and out of the car all day, in all weathers and I am coping nicely. Furthermore, on my last visit to my G.P. my blood pressure was normal, the lowest it has been for four years.

I have been lucky – I have a wife who cares for me, and gently persuaded me to do something about the health deterioration which she had observed in me. I knew something was wrong but initially easily found "good reasons" for feeling the way I did. Had I not been diagnosed with mild hypothyroidism and accepted the very simple and straightforward medication I would have been experiencing some serious health problems by now and would most certainly have a poorer quality of life.

KNOW your body: LISTEN to what it is telling you and DO something about it when you know all is not well.

MY OBSERVATIONS OF NORMAN:

I had always been aware of Norman's colouring, it had a yellowish tinge to it. One of the reasons could be that carotene was not being converted to Vitamin A because of the thyroid malfunction. His colouring is now normal.

His eyes sometimes looked very red and, when I asked him, he stated they were very sore. He was suffering from the "dry eye" syndrome. He is rarely affected by this condition now.

Dry skin was another sign and healing processes were much slower. He had a tendency to put on weight and sometimes a blank look as if it was taking forever for something to register.

Norman is in the best of health now and enjoys life much more with his new found energy and sense of well-being. He was on beta-blockers for high blood pressure. He no longer needs to take that medication as his blood pressure is now normal.

SUFFERERS WHO CONTACTED A HELPLINE IN MANCHESTER RUN BY CAROLINE HULME.

SUSAN – BOLTON
DIAGNOSED TREATED CASE OF HYPOTHYROIDISM: STILL NOT WELL.

After the results of a blood test for thyroid function, my doctor diagnosed hypothyroidism and prescribed a dose of 150 microgrammes of thyroxine per day. Since the initial diagnosis, I have had blood tests every six months. My daily amount of thyroxine had never been altered. There has been little improvement. However, I do not feel that the problem has been adequately addressed in so far as many of the symptoms still persist.

The tiredness is still excessive and debilitating: I am overly sensitive to heat and cold; the condition of my hair has not improved significantly; unpleasant palpitations occur from time to time. Most distressing of all is the frequent emotional over-sensitivity, mood swings, and mild depression. These persistent symptoms make the quality of daily life very poor. I can only assume that the persistence of these symptoms is due to under prescription of thyroxine.

ANNA – TAPORLEY
DIAGNOSED TREATED CASE OF HYPOTHYROIDISM: STILL NOT WELL.

I have been diagnosed for the last twenty years as suffering from anxiety and depression. I have had a huge array of symptoms during this period. Many tests and x-rays and the doctors always reached the same conclusion – there was nothing wrong.

Finally, in 1993, one doctor thought I could have a thyroid problem. This had never been aired before. So a sample of blood was sent for testing. The doctor wrote to say that my thyroid gland was under-active. I was so relieved and happy, at last they knew what was wrong after twenty years of suffering.

December 1993	Diagnosed hypothyroid.
January, 1994	Started thyroxine 25 microgrammes.
February, 1994	Blood test - medication up to 50 microgrammes.
March, 1994	Blood test - Doctor says, "You are o.k. you do not need any more thyroxine, you are euthyroid."

I cannot begin to tell you how ill I felt. I was much worse by September, 1994.

I was to remain on this small dose of thyroxine as two doctors in the surgery both declared that the blood test result showed that I did not need any more thyroxine, in spit of the fact that I felt so ill. I put on a further stone in weight. I then decided to take matters into my own hands. I know now – I knew then – that the doctors were quite wrong and I have proved that by the action I took, I upped the dose and I am feeling very well."

A missed case of hypothyroidism is one who has many signs and symptoms and is in the lower end of normal range of FT4 or FT3 blood test result.

Missed cases and diagnosed treated cases, who are not yet well, suffer in the same way. The next few pages will show what I mean. I have mixed the missed cases of hypothyroidism and the diagnosed treated cases of hypothyroidism to demonstrate this to you.

82

I suffered with fatigue, weight gain, hair loss, dry skin (used to be greasy), swollen feet, ankles, calves and hands. Phlegm in upper part of chest, sore throats, loose bowels, dizziness with rapid head movements, and an inability to refocus quickly, lumpy swallowing, poor finger-nails, concentration diminishing, spots, painful and stiff joints, skin allergies, little lumps on skin on back of hands and trunk front and back, palpitations, right ear popping and shushing, severe migraine, double/quad vision, fainting after swimming, loss of sense of purpose, frequent bouts of flu and cold with a slow recovery rate, I was diagnosed by a private G.P. as having an underactive thyroid.

> *This patient is now very well and has lost all the excess weight she had. Her energy level has returned to normal; also, her sense of purpose has returned.*

DOROTHY
TALKS ABOUT HER TWENTY-ONE-YEAR-OLD DAUGHTER JULIE : A MISSED CASE OF HYPOTHYROIDISM.

For the past two years my daughter has been complaining of tiredness. She has been gaining weight (sometimes she has a bloated look) and has very dry skin. She is always cold and wears day clothes in bed. Her hair has become thinner.

More recently she's been upset, saying she has a pain in her chest (even thinking she has heart trouble). She is constantly in pain.

About nine months ago, she presented these symptoms to our G.P., and a blood sample was sent to test for anaemia which proved to be fine. There was no thyroid test done. Her paternal grandmother had an over-active thyroid.

I was diagnosed with hypothyroidism in 1989 after a dreadful twelve months of not knowing what was wrong with me. The two classic symptoms of weight gain and hair loss are still with me after four years of treatment.

MARIAN –TYNESIDE
MISSED CASE OF HYPOTHYROIDISM

I am concerned that the public knows so little about the condition of hypothyroidism. Many are suffering for too long before it is diagnosed. I lost my job. The doctor wrote a letter saying that I was unwell due to the stresses of my work. I asked my G.P. whether I could see a psychologist because I could not understand why I was so depressed and listless. I saw him for many weeks and got precisely nowhere. At a later date, he said to me, "Have you got a thyroid problem?" My reply was that surely the G.P. would have found it if I had. I was diagnosed six months later.

One lady 'phoned Caroline in desperation because her husband had been put on 250 microgrammes of thyroxine straight away and one of his many side effects was that he was having chariot races in the early hours of the morning. He was very restless and was having panic attacks. She was very worried because he used to drive long distances but refused to go back to the doctors because, "they put him on the dosage and they know best."

A twenty-eight-year-old girl was told that she was on the menopause and was put on to H.R.T. After some time and many problems, a thyroid test was done that proved positive.

84

Calls to the helpline are frequently from, what the medical profession call, border-line cases, who feel extremely poorly but get no help from their doctors and are not even given the opportunity for a repeat blood test.

GILLIAN – SOUTH WALES
DIAGNOSED TREATED CASE OF HYPOTHYROIDISM:
STILL NOT WELL.

After being ill for some time without knowing what was wrong with me, my doctor sent a sample of blood to be tested primarily for cholesterol levels as my blood pressure was high. When the results came back, I was told my cholesterol level was fine but my thyroid was overactive. I did not show any of the classic symptoms of overactivity i.e. weight loss and hyperactivity.

In fact, over the last three months, my weight has increased by 3st and I was so tired with no energy to run round and do the chores.

I was referred to the hospital to see a consultant who confirmed the diagnosis and explained the options re treatment, either pills (not really recommended) or radio-active capsule. I opted for the capsule and was sent for a scan to gauge the dose. They also carried out an E.C.G. as my pulse rate was very high. I had put this and the palpitations down to anxiety.

The consultants in the Nuclear Medicine Department had a long talk with me after the scan and explained much more than the other doctor I had seen. A week later I had my capsule.

Two months later, I went for check up and had another blood test after which I was summoned back to the hospital in one month instead of the proposed three months. This time I saw another consultant and was told that the radio-iodine had worked too well and my thyroid was now underactive. I was started on 100 microgrammes of thyroxine per day. I mentioned, in my last visit, that

85

sometimes when I moved I became dizzy and could not focus properly. My G.P. advised me to go to the optician. The optician told me that I had double vision (hence not being able to focus properly) when I looked to the right and upwards. Apparently this was due to the thyroid and would correct itself once the thyroid had returned to normal with the thyroxine.

Neither my G.P. nor the hospital have any leaflets regarding this condition.

The last six months have been very worrying and somewhat scary. How soon will I start to feel well and function properly again? I had to leave my job because I felt so ill and did not know what the outcome would be. Since then, I have felt so feeble and pathetic, I have wondered if I will every feel well again.

KAREN – MANCHESTER
FINALLY DIAGNOSED TREATED CASE OF HYPOTHYROIDISM WHO, AFTER FIVE YEARS OF TREATMENT, IS STILL NOT WELL

For a long time I had been feeling unwell and paid many visits to the doctor's surgery. I told my G.P. of the many different symptoms I was suffering from but he said I looked all right. He gave me pain-killers for the pain I was experiencing in my muscles and joints.

I reached the stage when I felt really ill but didn't like going to the doctor because he made me feel that it was all in my head. I knew it wasn't. I felt dreadfully ill and I had no idea what it could be.

It was such a relief to find out that was wrong with me after all this time of feeling so ill.

I have been on thyroxine now for five years and I still suffer from tiredness, and low energy. I have trouble with my eyes. The muscles behind the eyes are weak and I get blurred vision. My legs are so weak I feel as though I am about to fall over. I experience muscle spasms in my legs at night. They start shaking and I have to wait until it stops. It is the most terrible sensation. I also have trouble with my bowels.

I keep going the best I can.

I developed an overactive thyroid when I was in my teens but after taking a radioactive iodine x-ray test I was told that I didn't need treatment.

When I was 29, I had a total hysterectomy and weighed 8 st 4 lbs. I stayed at that weight until I attended a three month check-up and was given a high dose of oestrogen. That was June 1980. By December 1980 I was nearly 12 st. I have been trying to lose weight since that date.

My other symptoms were water retention, bloating of the stomach, forgetfulness, hair thinning, dry skin, listlessness, my skin was sallow and I never felt well. I also had high blood pressure.

After many visits to my G.P. I was sent for kidney x-rays and scans for a gall bladder. I was told my kidneys were not working properly and treated with frusemide (40 mg a day). It reached the stage when after many visits, the doctors made me feel like a hypochondriac and that the symptoms were all in my head.

In recent months I have suffered from very high blood pressure and was told to rest.

I went to see a doctor privately who diagnosed hypothyroidism. He said the blood tests were not reliable enough.

In just two weeks my blood pressure dropped dramatically from 160/180 to 170/90. After being on treatment for a while I do not need the diuretics. My skin has lost its sallow appearance and I have more energy than I can ever remember.

I have had a thyroid condition since birth (I was born without a thyroid) and have been on medication since then. I have regular blood tests which are always returned with the result low and never normal. the doctors always want me to take extra tablets. I recently had a blood test and the doctor wrote to me stating that the level was too low. He advised that I take 200 microgrammes of thyroxine a day. This seemed too high for me.

Since then I have seen another doctor who told me that the dosage was too high, and he prescribed 50 microgrammes.

I feel I am not getting the proper treatment. I have asked to see a specialist but my doctor refuses to refer me.

CONCLUSION

The same stories keep emerging, the doctor says either they are neurotic or they are depressed. Of course they are, wouldn't anyone be depressed after years of feeling well below par?

Caroline started the helpline after her second child was born with thyroid aplasia. Aplasia is total or partial failure of development of an organ or tissue.

Caroline needed information and reassurance but there was none. Staff at the hospital told her to go away and forget it. Forget it! How could she? She had somehow to administer medication to her daughter every day until she was old enough to take it herself. Caroline was told her daughter would need medication for life. Her baby could not tell her how she was feeling. Was she on enough medication? So many questions but no answers! No one to talk to,. Nobody wanted to know. The truth was that nobody knew enough to be able to tell her anything useful.

Caroline was determined to find out more. She started the helpline armed with a couple of addresses from the health visitor.

In the first year she had fewer than six enquiries. This grew steadily over the years. In 1993/1994 she had around three thousand enquiries. Of all these enquiries 60% are not satisfied with their treatment and still do not feel well after years on medication. This is usually put down to mental anxiety. Many doctors prescribe antidepressants to alleviate these symptoms.

There is much ignorance about thyroid disorders and yet it really is so simple to treat. I am horrified that after twelve years of Caroline providing a helpline – NOTHING HAS CHANGED.

THE FOLLOWING STORIES ARE FROM FELLOW SUFFERERS WHO USED THE DIANA HOLMES HELPLINE

FIONA CAMPBELL – DENTIST

I had been treated for depression for approximately eight years. The medication was a subclinical dose of imiprimine, a tricyclic antidepressant. For years, tiredness and other symptoms were attributed to depression.

The greater problems began after the birth of my son, Alex, in February 1994.

Around three months after Alex was born, instead of gradually feeling better, my state of health declined.

I was constantly exhausted, to the point of being unable to sit down without falling asleep. I had a total lack of energy and motivation and dragged myself around.

My hair became thin, my skin excessively dry and the outer third of my eyebrows disappeared.

I had exercised routinely three or four times a week before becoming pregnant and a couple of times a week up to thirty-six weeks of my pregnancy. I restarted exercising six weeks after the birth. I breast-fed my baby and with that, together with exercising, I expected my weight to return to normal, but it slowly crept up and then increased dramatically when I stopped breast-feeding my baby at eight months.

My G.P. agreed that I showed symptoms of hypothyroidism. He repeated tests for anaemia, leukaemia, thyroid malfunction, adrenal insufficiency and pituitary disturbances which were all returned within the "normal range". At my request, my G.P. referred me to a consultant endocrinologist. He concluded that I had M.E. (Myalgic encephalo myelitis) and advised "total rest"!

As you can imagine this was impossible, with a dental surgery to run together with a staff of nine and a toddler at home.

I became disillusioned and resigned myself to the fact that I was fat and depressed and losing my hair and this was "my lot".

Then, quite by chance, I read an article in an old magazine at work about a lady who had contacted Diana and was now improving in health.

At the earliest opportunity, I 'phoned Diana and she asked me a long list of questions a frightening number of which I answered "yes" to. These questions drew my attention to a number of symptoms I had not previously associated with hypothyroidism. I had suffered with some of these symptoms for years.

Diana then sent me a stack of literature on the subject. I photocopied this and passed it on to my G.P. He was still pretty sceptical at this stage. He spoke, however to a professor of endocrinology, at Birmingham University, which seemed to reassure him.

After this, my G.P. prescribed thyroxine with a grave warning about side effects and that I was not to raise my hopes.

The initial dose was 25 micrograms. After two of three days I felt better. (I cautiously reminded myself that this could be psychosomatic!)

Gradually, over the first month, my energy levels returned. One drawback in the early stages was that with more energy I tried to do more and I ended up regressing. I remember that Diana did warn me about this.

I saw my G.P. after the first month and he was impressed, albeit a trifle dubious but he increased the thyroxine to 50 micrograms.

A blood test at this stage confirmed that the thyroxine was having a beneficial effect. I attended the G.P.'s surgery after another month and he noticed a marked difference in me again.

Some months later, I am nearly back to what I consider normal energy levels. I spend more time awake than asleep and have my life back again.

I am eternally grateful.

MAGGIE HARRISON'S STORY

Just a little insight in to my life as it was...

At the age of twenty six, I was divorced with three young children. This meant a lot of work; cooking, cleaning, all the other household chores plus gardening and decorating, all of which I managed quite well, as well as a part-time job. When the kids were old enough, I started working full time. I had a lot of friends and was happy with lots of energy and I used to giggle when people said, "I don't know how you do it."

I was in my late 30's when I lost my mum and dad. I took both their deaths very badly. At the age of thirty six, I had hot flushes and palpitation attacks. The G.P. I had at the time started me on H.R.T. He said I was starting the menopause. My life and my health were still pretty good.

My fortieth birthday I planned to celebrate in style and hired a hall. I did all the catering myself and my friends and family celebrated with me. I had noticed myself putting on a bit of weight but didn't worry too much. At 9 st 2 lbs I could afford to put on a little.

I didn't really notice my weight piling on but by the time I was forty two I weighed 11 st. I found this really hard to cope with and could not understand why I had put on so much weight. In the following years I started to have problems. My stomach was very painful and I went to the hospital a couple of times with this and received numerous diagnoses, including stress, muscular spasms in my intestines and more stress.

Eventually, I went to a homeopathic clinic and I was treated for an allergy to yeast and gluten. I found this very difficult when shopping, as nearly everything on the shelves contained either gluten or yeast. Other things began to happen and the weight piled on and on and then I stopped socialising. I couldn't bear my friends seeing me like this plus the fact that my energy was slipping. I felt exhausted mentally and physically. My muscles and bones ached. I started to become concerned. What was happening? Was it my age? or was it because I was going through the menopause.

I paid a few visits to the doctor's surgery and came out either holding a diet sheet or a prescription. Neither of them did I want or need. I just wanted someone to listen to me. I went to see a counsellor who taught me how to relax as I was stressed. He also said I had to learn to like myself before I could get well. By this time, at the age of forty seven, my weight had risen to 14 stone 2 lbs.

My body started to swell, also my face, neck, hands, legs and ankles. Fluid tablets were prescribed. I had to push myself hard to do certain chores. Those same chores I used to sail through at one time. I couldn't garden any more or vacuum. I was too exhausted even to get the vacuum out.

I knew it was not normal. I went on diet after diet. I even tried slimming pills and eventually, I changed my eating habits, no fats, low salt, brown bread, etc., but my weight was still piling on. In the meantime, I had been for four or five blood tests to test for low thyroid and each one came back "normal". Each time I heard the word "normal", I cried. I've cried a lot over the past few years. I was also beginning to get breathless and found it difficult to climb the stairs or do a lot of walking (which I used to love).

When my doctor checked me over I had developed high blood pressure and asthma. Both needed treatment. I thought maybe I would start to feel better but things got worse. Although I had a full time job and an important role at work I coped well but was physically exhausted. I seemed to be dragging myself from A to B. The exhaustion brought me to tears and of course the first thing that comes to the minds of G.P.s when they see tears are the words, "STRESS" or "DEPRESSION". If I had a pound for every time I have been diagnosed with one of these I would be a millionairess.

I had also developed the following symptoms; migraines, lower back pain (I had numerous visits to the chiropractor for my back), dry skin, soft nails, body overheating, breathlessness, panic attacks, fits of uncontrollable sobbing, poor concentration, claustrophobia, personality change, lack of confidence, dry mouth, hoarseness and loss of voice, muscle spasms in my legs and arms, my vision was blurred and I had constipation.

Some of the symptoms I did not tell the doctor, I did not want him to think he had a crazy person as a patient. I had begun to think half of these symptoms were in my head. I put most of them down to my weight, age and the menopause.

One day at work, one of my friends handed me a clipping about thyroid trouble from a magazine. I couldn't believe it when I read it and recognised the symptoms I had were actually in writing and someone had experienced the same horror as myself!

There was a 'phone number to contact and I did so right away. It took a few tries but eventually I got through and Diana answered. She was lovely and understood everything I was going through. "At last," I cried. "Someone believes me!" We had quite a few conversations and Diana gave me guidance on how to approach the G.P. with my illness.

Finally, I went to the doctor and spoke frankly about the thyroid, as my last blood test showed it to be sluggish enough for treatment. I tried so hard not to cry. I put my views to him and told him I didn't think it was fair that I should suffer in this way. I didn't believe the blood test, which had been taken five months previously. The doctor listened and decided on another blood test and an appointment with a "Thyroid Specialist". I felt quite enthusiastic about this. The blood test came back "NORMAL" yet again! I was so upset. The doctor gave me a photocopy of the results to show the specialist and he wished me luck and said, "Let's hope she starts you on thyroxine, so that you can be well again."

A few weeks later, my visit to the specialist came. She gave me a thorough examination from head to toe. She then chatted and asked about my symptoms. Then came the words, "We'll do another blood test." I couldn't be doing with all that waiting again. I told her I had photocopies of my last blood test and proceeded to give them to her. She checked them over and said, "That's the one. I am treating you as of today and you will start on thyroxine." She then went on to say that they have to be 101% sure of a patient needing this drug as it has to be taken for life. But I didn't care. My illness was not my imagination. I had finally been diagnosed as having thyroid trouble and the lump in my neck that was diagnosed as fatty tissue is a "Goitre".

I floated out of the hospital. Sounds silly but I was so happy. Seven years of hell and finally I had been diagnosed. The first person I 'phoned was Diana and she expressed great joy for me and seemingly, I was her eighth success.

I have only been on thyroxine for three weeks and I feel great. I know I've got a long way to go before I am back to normal but I thank the day my friend in the office handed me the clipping from the magazine. Thank you, Diana, if it weren't for you, I might not have fought so hard.

I was one of the lucky ones though, because for the last five years I've had a man who has stood by me through all my moods, tears and aches and pains. He has done all the chores I couldn't do, which was almost everything and he was always there for me.

SYLVIA HULLAH – CHESHIRE

"She was always tired"

Had I not read a short article about Diana and subsequently contacted her 'She was always tired' was surely destined to become my epitaph, for goodness knows, my family had heard it often enough.

I was, in fact, at home recovering from an operation, flicking through a pile of old magazines when I saw a photograph of an attractive, tanned woman and felt compelled to read on – why, I don't know, because I was only tearing out recipes and certainly had not stopped to read anything else. As I read Diana's account, I began to think 'this is me' always tired, migraine, weight gain etc., but surely I couldn't have an underactive thyroid because I had been tested for it at least twice and the results were normal. Nevertheless I cut out the article and dwelt on it for a few days. On June 7th, 1996, I telephoned Diana and felt an immediate *rapport*. Here was someone who understood what I meant by "the last dregs of energy seemingly being swept out of your body from the toes upwards and out of the top of your head, leaving you feeling utterly exhausted!" After a long chat, Diana suggested a meeting with Dr. Skinner.

MONDAY, 10TH JUNE, 1996: Visited my own G.P. and told her about the work being done by Diana and Dr. Skinner. I emphasised that while not wishing to offend her, I felt she had exhausted all avenues. She was happy for me to see Dr. Skinner and expressed an interest in the outcome.

WEDNESDAY, 12TH JUNE, 1996: Appointment with Dr. Skinner. Arrived late, following a motorway jam but thankfully appointments were over-running. Sat in the garden with Diana. I was impressed with her bubbly personality and apparent abundant energy – could this really be the person in the wheel-chair?

Dr. Skinner said he was virtually certain, simply by looking at me, that I was suffering from hypothyroidism. He suggested starting treatment and was delighted to know that my G.P. was willing to administer this. Left Dr. Skinner really elated – at last someone had listened, understood and felt the situation could be remedied. Spent the rest of the day walking on air.

Dr. Skinner had asked for a photograph of how I looked, prior to what I had now discovered were fairly reliable hypothyroid indicators, i.e. puffy eyelids, thinning eyebrows, etc. It was hard to find close-up photographs, as for some time I had been so embarrassed and repulsed by my excess weight and appearance that I tended to avoid the camera like the plague, much to the regret of my husband, a keen photographer.

It was while searching for these photographs, that it suddenly began to dawn on my husband and I just how long ago this had started to develop – we had to go back twenty years. It was then that I began to feel angry. I had battled with my weight while it crept slowly but inexorably from 8½ st to almost 18½ st; had tried numerous diets; attended various slimming clubs, all to no avail. Over the years I had spent a great deal on alternative therapies – acupuncture, homeopathy, hypnotherapy, reflexology, aromatherapy – clutching at straws. We even had a man with dowsing rods identifying lay lines and then hammering copper tubing into the ground to divert the energy, as I had heard a programme on the radio about the effects these could have on some people's energy levels. "Gosh," I can hear you say, "This woman's a nutter," to which I would have replied, "No, I'm not but I was desperate –I just wanted to feel well." I felt extremely angry at having to spend so many years relatively inactive and at the effect this had on family life. At not even having the energy to help fund raising for a local animal rescue society, a cause dear to my heart and one which I had been instrumental in getting off the ground; at being unable to go on bike rides with my children – years of frustration, time lost for ever.

EARLY JUNE 1996: Who am I? I am a lethargic, lack-lustre teacher in her early fifties with a wonderful husband, a twenty-five-year-old son, a twenty-three-year-old daughter and four cats.

Around about 1974/75, I recall visiting my G.P. complaining of tiredness, which was probably understandable to a degree with two small children to look after but also expressing dismay at my rapidly increasing weight. I think a thyroid function test was carried out at this time. I distinctly remember being told to "eat less and to join a slimming club," and when I countered with the comment that I did not eat a lot, being told, "My dear, there are no fat Biafrans," and was sent away with a flea in my ear.

During the next ten years, I soldiered on, having returned to my job in 1978. Throughout this time my weight was still a problem, migraine was becoming a fairly frequent occurrence and I was always tired. By early 1983, I had reached the stage where I was constantly tired, my joints ached, I often had a sore throat accompanied by thin blisters on the inside of my lips and I would suddenly forget what I was saying half way through a sentence. It had reached a stage where I was no longer able to do my job properly, I just wasn't doing justice to the students or myself. I felt ill but I didn't want to give up the job I loved, all I wanted was for my problems to be diagnosed and the appropriate treatment to be given.

I went back to my G.P. who by now had heard my tale of woe several times. I explained the situation so far as the school was concerned and asked him for a sick note. He refused! Why? Because he couldn't put a name to what was wrong with me but agreed that rest would probably help matters. I left the surgery on the verge of tears. What was I going to do? No sick note, no pay and too sick to teach effectively. We had recently moved house, taken on a larger mortgage and I could ill afford to forego what ultimately turned out to be half a year's salary.

I was away from school from Easter until September and I must admit I returned feeling much better. I had believed, wrongly, as it would now appear, that I was suffering from glandular fever. In fact, I have been labouring under that impression for the last thirteen years or so and structured my life to fit in with this debilitating ailment.

Around the mid-eighties, I was transferred to my present lady doctor within the same practice. By now, the symptoms were well established – extreme tiredness accompanied by inability to sleep, continued weight gain, etc. She repeated the thyroid test – result normal and then proceeded to do all the other tests she could think of. By now my resistance was so low, I caught everything that was going. After all, schools are not the healthiest of places in which to work. School holidays were spent resting as much as possible in order to get fit enough to face the next term.

Three years ago I became involved in the delivery of the G.N.V.Q. course. In teaching circles, those dreaded initials have become synonymous with stress. In an attempt to help with the tiredness and possibly engender a feeling of well-being, my G.P. prescribed H.R.T. Great I thought, I'll be like Margaret Thatcher, bags of energy with a razor sharp mind and with the possibility of all the other benefits, beautiful skin, shining hair and strong nails. I willingly stuck on the patches. Of course, I was aware of the other side of the coin, possible weight gain but quite honestly I had reached the stage of even being prepared to accept that if in exchange I was also the recipient of the benefits of this elixir of life. Well did I get the pluses? No, I did not but I certainly got the minuses with a vengeance – almost three stone of it.

By now, excessive weight had taken its toll on my feet and I developed osteo-arthritis. Walking anywhere but the shortest distances was becoming increasingly painful. Walking on hard surfaces felt like walking on broken glass. Outings were very much determined by the proximity of car parking facilities. And yes, you've guessed it, even less exercise meant more weight gain; more weight, deteriorating feet, the proverbial vicious circle. To say I didn't walk for pleasure would not be exactly true. My caring sympathetic husband thought that maybe walking on the beach would be more comfortable and so we would drive to Llanudno, a round trip of about 120 miles so that I could walk for possibly half an hour. In February 1995 I had the first of three operations on my feet.

Despite extreme tiredness, sleep, especially high quality sleep, evaded me. I was up every morning at 5 a.m. (Saturday and Sunday included) even though I didn't need to leave home until 8.15 a.m. I began to experience alarming visual distortion. If I moved my head rapidly, it was almost as though my eyes were a split second behind in focusing on the new aspect. Equally disconcerting was the inability to retain any new information. As a teacher, I had always prided myself on being able to learn and remember pupils' names, usually within the first one hour lesson. Suddenly this was no longer the case. How could I account for this? I told myself it was probably due to the increased work load, but deep down I was becoming increasingly worried by this new and unfamiliar phenomenon. A few years ago, my father died of Alzheimer's' disease and this was one of the first apparent signs that all was not well. I kept these fears to myself.

By January 1996, I had reached rock bottom. My feet were agony, climbing the stairs made me breathless, I was struggling to keep my head above water. Early retirement, on grounds of ill health, seemed to be the only sensible course of action. The wheels were set in motion.

I am pleased to say that throughout this time, while health diminished, vanity did not. I have always loved clothes and because I made most of my own, I was thankfully able to give myself a psychological boost. Even though I changed from my original size 12 up to 22, for most of the time I used a size 14 pattern and cut it out larger. It was really only when I became so exhausted and no longer had the energy to make my own, that I then found myself seeking out the 16 and over shops and having to buy size 22 or 24. However, not to be defeated, as soon as I got home I cut out the label. Inside this fat body there has always been a slim person.

Now I look forward to the day when I don't care if the label sticks out! I'd be proud to announce to the world, look at me, I'm size 14 again.

- **19th March, 1996:** Second foot operation.
- **3rd May, 1996:** Third foot operation – that makes it sound as though I have three feet, I haven't.
- **18th June, 1996:** After my visit to Dr. Skinner he wrote to my G.P. who in turn carried out a further thyroid function test and promised to start thyroxine treatment when the result was received. I literally counted the hours until my next appointment. My poor long suffering husband was now faced with something akin to the speaking clock – 85 hours to go, 47 hours to go, 31 hours to go, until eventually 9 hours to go, down to single figures at last.
- **7th June, 1996:** Test result received – NORMAL. Thyroxine treatment started.
- **July, 1996:** Who am I? Well, to be absolutely frank, I am not sure. I'm certainly not me, not the me I've known for the last few years especially. I find it hard to recognise this energetic, lively, organised person, willing to take on whatever is thrown at her. My

colleagues can't believe it. They are amazed at the transformation. I find it incredible that the test was NORMAL.

I am still on a low dose of thyroxine. Diana informed me that I've a long way to go yet. I simply cannot believe it, it feels as though I've leapt straight from the early seventies straight through to the mid-nineties and the intervening period was all a bad dream.

Reading about and meeting Diana has been far better than winning the lottery. After all, had I won the lottery, what would I be doing now? I'd probably be house hunting in France, buying size 22 designer clothes and masses of shoes and still saying "Why am I so tired, why can't I lose weight and, oh no, here comes another migraine..."

Diana, I admire your courage and tenacity in pursuing your mission. It can't be easy and no one would have blamed you if, when finally having resolved your own situation, you had turned round and said, "Now I am going to get on with my life and make up for all those lost years."

P.S. Tomorrow I am going to buy a bike!

IMELDA'S STORY – TAKEN FROM HER DIARIES

1989: Polycystic ovarian disease - periods stopped after pill – clomiphene given –produces periods – no pregnancy.
1991 Sept. Hospitalised – hyperstimulation of ovaries – very ill – PREGNANT.
1992: Very difficult pregnancy – Alicia born May – periods return, very heavy – 4 weekly (this is new to me).
1993 Sept: Very tired – drained – aches and pains in arms and legs. Pins and needles in hands and feet. Everywhere feels tight and swollen. Period irregular – cannot keep track – gone off course.
1993 Dec: Waking up with numb hands.
1994 Jan: Carpal Tunnel Syndrome – visit G.P. – rest.

101

1994 Feb: Very bad headache – no period.

1994 Mar: Fatigue – run down – weight gain

1994 April: Fat but can't stop eating.

1994 May: Feel period wants to start.

1995 Mar: Hands swollen – pins and needles in feet – feel heavy.

1995 April: Big toe – numb, can't feel the top – this frightens me.

1995 May: Balance slightly off – feel panicky – left leg making me trip up.

1995 July: Left leg feels as if it is not there –numb below knee.

1995 Aug: Have a hormonal headache – bad.

1995 Sept: Can't get up – joints aching – eyes very bad with pins and needles – it's like a screwdriver being driven through them. This lasted 3 weeks. G.P. says TENSION!

1995 Oct: Have a bad throat – can't swallow. Back of ankles painful. Can't get warm. Heels and arches under feet hurting. I have palpitations – left leg muscle constricted and burning. I AM VERY ILL AND VERY FRIGHTENED! Diagnosis- Fobromyalgia.

1995 Nov: Feel a bit better – antidepressants make me feel worse.

1995 Dec: Christmas Day neck being attacked – squeezed – agitated –itching – burning – red rash across front going up towards my ears. It feels like two fingers being pushed into where the Adam's apple is.

1996 Jan: Neck still red and itching – then feels like daggers being aimed at the front of my neck. Take aspirin – very painful.

1996 Feb: Doctors say I have arthritis in my neck – given a leaflet.

1996 Mar: Palpitations – feel like I am ready to take flight – heart pounding –breathless – imagining terrible things – can't concentrate – balance affected - cannot read stories to my little girl – speech slurs – words get mixed up.

1996 April: Doctors still quoting, "Play about with the tricyclic drugs" (antidepressants). Taken Dothiepin – have to stop as I am becoming a zombie. Have not had a blood test since last October. G.P. decides to test me for Cushing's disease – result normal. G.P. will not test for thyroid. As far as he is concerned I have Fibromylagia.

1996 May: I read an article about Diana in *Woman* magazine. I had to push myself to ring Diana. I was so desperate. I was sure that people thought I was making a meal of the Fibroymyalgia. Symptoms came and went or were there altogether.

1996 June 5th : See Diana at last and Dr. Skinner. Feel like we are speaking the same language. Now taking thyroxine – after five days – no palpitations – no breathlessness – co-ordination back – less panicky – mind has stopped rushing – cloud has risen. The volume is being turned down on my symptoms – left leg is normal – I COULD CRY UNTIL MY G.P. says that thyroxine is like L.S.D. and will give a buzz especially if you believe in it – felt like piggy in the middle. My eyes are movable again. The only symptom left is the pain in my shins like screws.

Imelda now has a much better quality of life.

MARTHA ROBERTS – WREXHAM

A Retired Deputy Head, Martha suffered with an overactive thyroid – aged 46 years – and received radio-active iodine treatment. Here is her story:

Here is an account of my thyroid troubles from the onset to a successful conclusion over thirty years ago. Looking back, it was a long struggle but the joy of "living again" is beyond belief. From that, "recovery" takes on a new meaning, life becomes a bonus and you thank God for giving you the will power to carry on through the dark days. Good health will never be taken for granted again.

103

In 1964, when still working for the Red Cross, I began to lose weight rapidly (2lbs a week). Although eating more heartily than usual, I was constantly hungry, my brain was working overtime and there was an urgency in all my activities. My heartbeat increased rapidly and I was hot and clammy. The feeling of cold sweat on my cheeks is clear to me now.

I developed a tremble which was only perceptible to me at first (a tremble in my flesh) but soon became apparent when I could not pour a cup of tea or pass a cup of liquid to someone.

My hair became dry and unmanageable and I lost my eyebrows. The obvious sign of an overactive thyroid, which was not noticeable at the time, was bulging eyes. I may have had deep set sockets so a little protrusion may not have shown and certainly did not interfere with my eyelids. I did have difficulty focusing but as my eyesight was not impaired I did not take it too seriously. Thankfully, I was able to find comfort and escape in reading.

As the condition worsened, I became very exhausted; my heart-beat was obvious as my head nodded with its severity. It was more noticeable when I lay down and often, at about 3 a.m., I would be frightened by a choking bout. I was so ill I could not deny it or hide it. Friends did not recognise me. I wanted to hide away. I lost interest in activities and personal contacts. I'd go to my room just to be alone. Activity, communication and infection (even the common cold) increased the palpitations until they became almost unbearable. I still craved for food and this excess increased my bodily functions.

I did have one great pleasure (besides eating). I loved going out in the car with my parents. The car was cosy and intimate and the engine noise masked my racing heart and I relaxed with loved ones who understood. I realise now what an anxious time it was for my parents. My dear mother told me, years later, that she feared I would die in the car as I looked so ill.

I am going to digress and tell you of an incident which happened when I was recovering. My friend took me to Port Talbot to stay with her cousin, whom I knew well so it was no great strain. At bedtime they apologised for the all-night noise from the steelworks and hope that it would not prevent me from sleeping. To me it was music for it masked my heavy rapid heart-beat and I slept all night, to their suprise.

Back to Easter 1965 when I had to face reality and give in as I was exhausted. Everything happened so quickly. I was in need of urgent attention and saw a specialist privately and he referred me to a specialist in Christie's Hospital, Manchester. Had I gone through the National Health it would have taken six weeks in those days for the thyroid blood test to be returned. I went to Christe's not knowing if my condition was due to an overactive thyroid or an even more serious condition that had not been diagnosed.

When I went to Christie's, I was given radio-active iodine to drink through a straw. I was not to touch the container and so kept my hands behind my back. When I had drunk it all I had to flick the cardboard container down a chute. The lady who gave it to me was sitting behind a glass panel as in a railway ticket office.

Then I was allowed to go out and have a meal in the hospital and was to return in the afternoon.

Back at Christie's in the afternoon, I was taken to have the test with the Geiger counter (this was to be the moment of truth which I prayed would be positive so that I could be treated). After the examination, I was taken to a room and told that I had an overactive thyroid which could be treated. I can see the room and the lady doctor now and feel the relief that I had had nothing worse. Little did I realise that it would take two-and-a-half years for my broken body to recover fully after the offending amount of thyroid was destroyed. It was a very slow process and the body had to recover at its own pace. Nature is slow but sure.

Slowly my interests were revived. I was pleased to see friends and to visit them. From then on I have tried to keep my priorities in the right order. I value and cherish normal life and especially children and people and the joy they give. Once again I could hear a babbling brook and hear the cows as they chewed the cud and how wonderful to hear the daffodils as they tinkled away in the breeze instead of a heavy loud racing heart.

I am humbly grateful for the wonderful blessings I have been privileged to receive.

There was one frightening set-back just when I had recovered sufficiently to enjoy life but hadn't the staying power to cope with full-time work. It was convalescent time which can be hard to handle. It must have taken me two years to reach this stage in my recovery. The set-back happened suddenly when I was feeling particularly well and had enjoyed a picnic. I was on top of the world.

I was on my way home when I had a strange feeling of not being "with it". I thought I was going to faint but I couldn't shake it off. To be honest, I thought I was going to die, I felt so dazed. When I arrived home I sat close to the fire to get warm (it was a warm day) and had some brandy to revive me. From then on I became lethargic, my knees were swollen and I put weight on. I found it difficult to walk. I had no idea what was happening to me. I was so disappointed.

I went to see Mrs Cole, the specialist from Christie's who had attended me throughout my illness. She was most apologetic and said, "Oh, I am sorry, you have become underactive. It does happen sometimes but we can put it right with tablets which you will have to take for the rest of your life."

I took the thyroxine and began to improve. It was a matter of months before I was back to normal again. Taking a dose of thyroxine every day is not problem.

The wonderful day arrived when I was discharged from hospital.

Shortly afterwards, I visited my G.P. He made me realise just how ill I had been. He went on to say, "Martha, it's a miracle, you could have died at any time," and clicked his fingers to emphasise the point. No wonder he had been advising me to retire but I was adamant that I was going back to work.

I was so happy to return to my work as a school teacher. I remember the joy (and a little trepidation) of going back to school. Even buying the daily paper on my way was memorable. Meeting the staff, pupils and parents was like a dream come true. I was surrounded by love and showered with bunches of flowers from true friends who shared my happiness.

I went back to work knowing that the rest of my life was a bonus to be treasured. I fulfilled my post as deputy head (having refused the headship) for the next ten years until my retirement in 1976. I was privileged to be given a wonderful but very emotional retirement get together by the whole school, parents and friends. I am humbly grateful and thank God.

Since my retirement, I have lived a very active life and had great happiness.

MARY EATON – OSWESTRY

I attended a medical practice in Oswestry.

The start of my health problems was twenty-six years ago. I had started to bleed heavily from my vagina. My legs were full of aches and pains. I made routine visits to my G.P. which, in the end, were fruitless as she said, "There's nothing wrong with you, you are too young to have anything seriously wrong with you." I lost weight rapidly and I was a deathly pale colour. This continued for a while. I met someone I had not seen for some time who was totally shocked at my appearance and immediately took me to hospital. In the end I had to have an emergency hysterectomy and blood transfusions. I was very poorly and all my G.P. got was a reprimand.

107

Almost six years later, I started to feel unwell and extremely tired with pains in my chest. Routine visits to the doctor's surgery, again, proved fruitless. Time went by and at one stage I was taken into hospital and put into intensive care and diagnosed with angina.

I had to give up work and was in and out of Shrewsbury and Stock hospital. I had very many tests and was attached to various machines including heart monitors.

I had signs and symptoms including weight increase, loss of hair, coarse hair, skin like leather, brittle nails, I lost hair from my eyebrows and my eyelashes fell out. I suffered for the next two years and my pulse rate became dangerously low.

I was taken to Stoke hospital. On the ward, I was surrounded by doctors and trainee doctors all scratching their heads as to what might be the matter with this twenty eight year old woman.

A young trainee doctor asked, "Has anyone tested for a thyroid problem?" No, was the answer. I was at the end of my tether. A blood test proved I had a thyroid condition.

Over the two years I had taken various medications and concoctions, all of which proved totally irrelevant to my condition. It appeared that all I needed was thyroxine. This was introduced very slowly until I was on 200mcgs daily which was to last for seventeen years. Two and a half years ago, my new G.P. reduced the thyroxine by 50cmgs as she was concerned that I might manifest signs and symptoms of an overactive thyroid. I showed no sign of being overactive at that time.

In March, 1988, the lymph nodes in my neck were very swollen and the family pressed me to return to the G.P. and seek his advice. The G.P. advised a biopsy.

I went in to hospital as a day-case. When I came around from the operation, I suffered excruciating pain in my neck and right shoulder. I was told that I must expect some discomfort after minor surgery. No one was interested. I was in agony. My arm swelled like a balloon and the pain continued. I returned to my G.P. who said, "There is nothing wrong, it will get better. Give it time."

My right shoulder dropped six inches and the muscles on the right side of my back were wasted away. I had an appointment to see the specialist. He found that the nerve that served the trapezious muscle had been damaged during the operation. I was devastated! I was paid compensation.

I rejoined the work-force although I still had aches and pains and my bones were becoming so painful. I thought at one time that maybe I had cancer of the bone.

I made yet another visit to the G.P. and had various tests of all which were negative.

So far I had been diagnosed with:

1. Angina.
2. Osteo-arthritis.
3. Spondylosis.
4. Ankylosing spondylosis.
5. Neurotic hypochondria.
6. Depression.
7. Bordering on psychosomatic tendencies.
8. Attention seeking.

Two and a half years ago, I moved home and had to change to a new G.P. in Oswestry and his attitude to me was rude to say the least. I changed my doctor, yet again, and moved to a different practice in Oswestry.

My symptoms now included constipation, panic attacks, exhaustion, hot flushes and chest pains.

I visited my new G.P., who appeared to believe what I was telling her. Many tests were carried out which all proved negative.

Approximately six months ago, I had a tooth extraction and needed two courses of antibiotics to clear away some infection which the dentist believed was due to a circulatory problem and he advised me to see my doctor immediately.

I had my eyes tested recently and there was no change and yet from time to time my eyes became blurred and I couldn't see. The optician had a good look at my eyes and asked if I was tired, to which I replied, "Yes." I told him I was hypothyroid and he urged me to go back to the doctor.

I told my G.P. everything. She listened but I don't think she heard me. She just sent me away.

I contacted Diana Holmes on her helpline. I decided to see a private consultant. I am terrified in case he finds nothing! Is it all in my head? I know I am getting worse. I am so tired and my energy levels are very low. I cannot stand heat now. I don't recognise myself. I know my body and I am not well. Please, God, let somebody help me because I cannot take much more. I have had to put up with being labelled a hypochondriac. In my notes at the G.P. it stated that, "I like visiting the doctor."

I am so angry and I am trying not to let bitterness take over but I feel so vulnerable and the very people I am supposed to trust have been indescribably negligent towards me. I still find it hard to believe all that has happened to me. I feel so hurt and raw inside. Without my faith and family I would have given up long ago. My G.P. says I enjoy all this.

I made an appointment with the private consultant – Dr. Gordon Skinner. After my consultation with Dr. Skinner, he increased my medication and said, "If you get the chance to see an endocrinologist, please do so."

I did get the chance to see an endocrinologist who was totally unprofessional. He stated I was middle aged and I should expect to put on weight and that some women wanted to take extra thyroxine to lose weight. He wanted to know who increased my thyroxine. I told him. "Dr. Skinner," he replied. "He's just a quack, he'll take your money and tell you what you want to hear. He's only interested in the cash." He said all this without even checking up on Dr. Skinner. Then he said, "I work for the

N.H.S." to which I replied, "I want someone working for me.

I am feeling so much better regarding my thyroid condition since Dr. Skinner increased my dose of thyroxine.

I am still plagued by a pain under my right breast. My G.P. said, "You have got to accept your illness and get on with your life. We have a number of ladies in the surgery who are obsessed with their body and their health. You cannot go on having tests, there is nothing life-threatening. You are your own worst enemy. You just sit at home." I told him the pain was like an ulcer that I had suffered years earlier. Begrudgingly he gave me a prescription for some losec. Unfortunately, this disabling pain is still with me and Dr. Skinner is doing all he can to help.

DEBORAH'S STORY, RELATED BY HER MOTHER ,BETTY.

Debbie was 40 years old when she died, unexpectedly, on January 19th, 1995, from a heart attack. One of the central aspects of Debbie's story is that she was, like many others, diagnosed treated and yet *still not well.*

Debbie's heart and arteries had been damaged as a result of her thyroid condition. She was not aware that her heart had been so badly affected, although ever since she had been diagnosed as hypothyroid, in May 1993, she had been concerned about damage to her heart and arteries. Not one member of the medical profession that she came in contact with in the last eighteen months of her life, took her fears seriously

Debbie was happily married and in 1984 became pregnant, much to our joy. When I saw Debbie I was immediately concerned because she did not look like a "blooming mother-to-be" but at three months it was still early days.

In February, 1985, Debbie had an instinctive feeling that something was wrong. She had had more than one scan and was told everything was all right, but she still felt

111

all was not well. At one ante-natal clinic it was discovered that the baby was dead and she had been carrying the dead foetus for two to three weeks, may be longer. She was taken into hospital immediately and given a "D & C". Within a matter of days, Debbie returned to work, hardly giving herself time to recover physically or grieve for the loss of her baby.

Following the loss of the baby, Debbie began to have weight problems and started to attend the Well Woman Clinic at her surgery. She was always "healthy eating", conscious of her problem and never indulged in junk food. However, she just did not seem to respond to diets, no matter how hard she tried at each regime.

We only saw Debbie two or three times a year during the twenty years she lived in London. She came for weekend visits sometimes accompanied by her husband. They both came to us for Christmas 1992 and Chris (Debbie's father) and I were very concerned to see Debbie looking tired and very overweight. At that time, she was attending a Well Woman Clinic and being weighed regularly.

Debbie and her husband were going to Spain for Easter and asked us if we would like to join them. We went down to London to join them for the day we were due to fly to Spain. We could not believe the dramatic change in Debbie – her body, face and hands were swollen and she had blisters on the palms. She looked a very unhealthy colour. Her hair had thinned so much, the outline of her skull was clearly visible.

She was also complaining of pain and discomfort in her limbs and had been to her G.P. because she feared she was suffering from rheumatoid arthritis like her father. A sample of blood was taken to test for rheumatoid arthritis but she had to wait two weeks for the result.

Chris has had rheumatoid arthritis and has been hypothyroid for thirty years and can no longer walk or stand. I could understand Debbie's fear of developing her father's condition but the more I looked at her the more I was convinced that she had a thyroid problem.

As well as a rheumatoid arthritis test Debbie was also tested for cholesterol and E.S.R. (Estimated Sedimentation Rate) but not a thyroid test. These tests came back negative. Debbie, of course, was relieved but still felt very unwell. I suggested she contact her G.P. on her return and arrange for a thyroid blood test. I don't think this registered with her but on her return home her friend Pat sent her a pamphlet about hypothyroidism and this finally convinced her this must be the cause of her feeling so ill.

She went to see her G.P. for another cholesterol test because they appeared to have lost the first one! She had listed her signs and symptoms although it was obvious just from looking at her that she had a thyroid problem. The G.P. agreed that she must be hypothyroid and we presume she carried out a thyroid function test although there was no record of this in her medical notes.

I felt a sense of relief because I know that hypothyroidism can be controlled by taking thyroxine. Chris has been diagnosed thirty years before following viral pneumonia which damaged his thyroid gland. He was started on a low dose – 25 micrograms increasing every month until he was on 200 mcgs, which, much later, was reduced to 150mcgs. Even with all the problems that Chris has had over the years, his heart is still undamaged.

Once the G.P. had established Debbie's hypothyroidism she started on a top dose of thyroxine – 100mcgs. Debbie took this amount for two to three days and started to feel very ill. She became agitated and was suffering from what she thought was a panic attack. She complained of a burning sensation throughout her body. The emergency doctor was called and he assessed her condition and advised her to stop taking the thyroxine and make another appointment with her G.P. after the weekend. He sedated her and left her enough tablets for the Sunday until she could make an appointment with her G.P. on Monday. Debbie saw her G.P. on Monday and

113

complained about the panic attack but there was no record of this in her medical notes or the fact that an emergency doctor had attended her on the Saturday evening.

The G.P. said that Debbie seemed unwell so she decided to restart her on a lower dose of thyroxine and built it up gradually.

Debbie responded to the thyroxine. There was an immediate weight loss. Her hair started to regrow, the blisters began to disappear and the puffiness in her hands and face was reduced. The next three months her mood swings continued to disturb her. She became more and more depressed and started to have obsessive thoughts about what damage a cholesterol level of 18.8 had done to her body. She talked about fears of having damaged arteries. This, of course, put stress on her marriage.

Debbie was finally referred to an endocrinologist four-and-a-half months later, by which time her cholesterol levels had returned to within normal limits. The consultant seemed satisfied with her diagnosis and progress and arranged to see her again in six months time.

She continued to get more depressed, stressed and anxious. She needed some answers, as to why she continued to fell unwell.

Debbie continued teaching but had a discussion with her head of department and told him how concerned she was that she wasn't functioning on all cylinders because of her thyroid condition.

In November 1993, Debbie went on an educational trip to Paris even though she was not really well enough. The length of stay was three days. On the evening of the third day, Debbie experienced another panic attack, similar to the one where the emergency doctor had been called out four months earlier.

Upon returning home, Debbie told her husband what had happened. He said their marriage was over. The rejection was too much for Debbie; she went into a complete state of hysteria. She had called us to tell us what had happened to her in Paris and her husband's reaction.

114

She then started to express suicidal thoughts. We knew our daughter needed help and had no choice but to call our other daughter Philippa, who was working and living in London at that time.

Philippa found it very hard to believe what we were telling her. She promised to leave work as soon as possible to help her sister. In the meantime, I kept ringing Debbie up every half hour or so until Philippa reached her. I wanted to hop on a train to London myself, but couldn't because Chris was still quite ill with a bad dose of 'flu. Philippa arrived in Kingston, helped pack some of Deb's clothes and then took her to a counsellor. The girls then went back to Philippa's flat in Fulham and somehow managed to get through the night with Debbie in a terrible state of shock.

Debbie's distress over the break up of her marriage reached an even greater level and Philippa took her back to Kingston to her own G.P. who prescribed sleeping tablets and said time would heal the pain.

At a later date, a psychiatric registrar assessed Debbie and agreed that she was suffering from severe reactive depression and needed to be admitted for treatment.

Debbie was to undergo further stress when her husband filed for divorce.

In November, 1994, Debbie started to work for the Terence Higgins Trust on a voluntary basis.

Now looking back to December 1994 I remember how tired she used to be after exertion. The pressure in her head was always there and seemed to become stronger in the evenings. She talked about her situation and her fears for the future and I did my best to reassure her.

There was a programme on the television about heart problems and all her old fears returned that there might be damage to her heart and arteries. I reassured her that the doctors would have diagnosed a heart condition had she had one. I suggested she have a check-up with her G.P. on her return home. This she did but only her emotional state was discussed.

115

We now know that she didn't ever feel strong enough to cope physically. Everything was such an effort for her but all of these feelings were put down to her depressive illness.

Debbie had been staying with Philippa for a few days. She called Philippa at her office and asked could she stay one more night. Philippa had arranged to go out but Debbie had her own key and had planned to watch T.V. once she returned from the cinema.

We had, over the last year, been in the habit of speaking to the girls every day. We rang Debbie to reassure her how much we loved her.

That night I rang her about 10.30 p.m. and I handed the 'phone to Chris, usually he used to call over to her and say goodnight but for some reason I thought it would be nicer if he spoke to her that night.

They talked for about ten minutes and then I spoke to her again reassuring her about going back to the flat the next day. She said she didn't need to get up so early, so I told her I would call her about 10 a.m. We said our usual goodnights but I knew that there was an urgency in her voice when she said, "I love you very much, mum. I love you very much, dad." I said, "We love you too, darling," with a feeling of puzzlement. We finished our conversation about 11 p.m. Philippa arrived home at about 12 p.m. She went into the lounge to find Debbie asleep on the sofa, tucked under her duvet – the T.V. was still on but in order not to disturb her because she looked in a deep sleep, she tiptoed across the room and switched it off.

At about 7 a.m. the next morning, Philippa got up and had a bath – even read a few pages of a book while having a soak, which was unusual for her to do so early in the day. She had a strange feeling, while drying her hair, that Deb was dead. There was something about the atmosphere in the flat that made her follow her instincts. She walked into the lounge and froze on the spot. Deb was lying in the same position as she had been the night before – as if she were in a peaceful sleep. She touched her sister – she was dead.

Philippa called the emergency services. The police and the ambulance arrived. Debbie's body was taken to the mortuary where a full post mortem was to take place. There had to be an autopsy to find the cause of death. The coroner was speedy with his response, he called us by noon the following day to tell us our daughter had died of a heart attack! This had never entered our heads – apparently she had had two minor heart attacks during the previous two years and there was cerebral damage – she could have had a stroke at any time and her thyroid gland was completely shrivelled up.

I personally find it incredible that this happened. Debbie came into contact with so many doctors and her heart condition was not diagnosed.

This is the danger once depression has been diagnosed, that all her symptoms of pressure in the head and tiredness are thought to be related to the depression and no further investigation is made. The real condition is masked and doctors agree that this does happen.

I subsequently spoke to all Deb's doctors, G.P.'s and consultants, a few weeks following her death. I was told more than once that sudden death happens for no apparent reason.

This was not the case with Debbie. There was a very good reason why her heart was damaged.

I was also told that she had said nothing to doctors that led them to believe that she had a damaged heart. Surely a cholesterol level of 18.8 should have warranted some investigation!

It seems to me that she was expected to do a self-diagnosis but even when she expressed her fears, nobody listened to her. They were all dismissed as obsessional thoughts.

Deborah grieved for her lost marriage every single day but because of her malfunctioning thyroid that was

117

possibly not being properly addressed, she did not have the physical stamina to overcome it.

She had been such a lovely, lively girl with sparkling eyes, who loved people – her students – her teaching – her cats – her home – her garden – her life!

My sincere hope is that other women should not slip through the net. I hope that Well Woman clinics are made aware of women who do not respond to diets and whose appearance changes so dramatically.

I hope that Deborah's story will at least prevent the same kind of tragedy happening again. The two photographs reproduced here convey something of the dreadful changes that occur during the onset of illness, and I know that she would have wanted you to compare them. On the left we see Debbie in 1993, overweight and presenting all the signs of myxodema before her treatment. On the right we see the beautiful and vivacious Debbie of 1988, before her illness, as we shall always remember her. God bless you, Debbie.

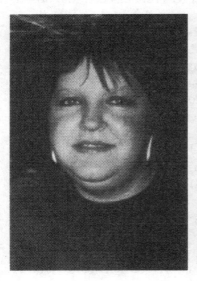 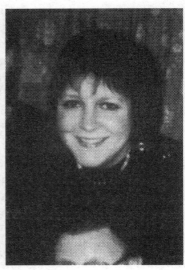

CHAPTER ELEVEN

WHAT IS HAPPENING OUT THERE?

When a G.P. first suspects a thyroid malfunction he sends a sample of the patient's blood to the laboratory for testing. If the result is returned "normal range", **even in the face of outstanding evidence to the contrary, the G.P. will revoke his initial diagnosis.**

Whatever happened to good old fashioned signs and symptoms, history and clinical appraisal? The doctor now diagnoses the blood test instead of the patient. The blood tests are good but should only be used as an indicator!

The role of patient and doctor seems to have been reversed. Instead of the patient telling the doctor how he/she feels the doctor now tells the patient that, if their blood test is returned in the normal range then there is nothing wrong.

How many times do you hear people say that upon entering the surgery the doctor is sitting there with the prescription pad in his/her hand?

Let us look at the words DOCTOR and PHYSICIAN. It doesn't matter which one we use. Both mean specialists in medical diagnosis and treatment.

Patients with diagnosed thyroid problems are not now diagnosed by the doctor or even have their treatment managed by a doctor because biochemists have taken over as diagnosticians.

Are we partly to blame?

One thing a doctor is afraid of is **litigation.** Everywhere you turn somebody is suing somebody. So those little words, on the blood test result slip, "normal range" are something for the doctor to hold on to.

Many patients, with the signs and symptoms set out in chapter seven, are told that they are depressed. The doctor prescribes antidepressants. Failing that it's either a virus, your age, or you are neurotic.

Here are some of the comments made to patients by doctors, bearing in mind that these patients are suffering with many signs and symptoms.

From G.P. or Consultant to Patient!

1. *"Take these tablets and you'll feel fine."* The doctor gave no explanation! No help! No guidance! The poor lady had just found out that she had an underactive thyroid and found herself outside the doctor's surgery with her mind in a whirl. She was left clueless and afraid.

2. Some doctors can be quite brutal. One lady was told, *"You are a hypochondriac."*

3. Patient to G.P. *"Can I have my thyroid checked?"* G.P. to patient, *"Oh, have you come up with something else now?"*

The next one is a classic:

4. *"The blood test dictates that you only need 50mcgs."* When the patient told me this, I had a mental image of little blood samples running around giving out orders.

Here's a few more:

5. *"At your age what do you expect?"*

6. A patient with over fifty signs and symptoms was told, *"It's wear and tear. You should be grateful you are alive."*

7. *"Come back when you've got cancer."*

8.   One patient with over sixty signs and symptoms asked her doctor would he do a thyroid function test and he refused.

Another patient is totally confused:

9.   One doctor tells her she is taking too much thyroxine, another tells her she is not taking enough.

This one is priceless:

10.   *"I just read the blood tests. I don't know anything about the thyroid."*

11.   A few patients on thyroxine therapy are on doses of more than 200mcgm as their optimum dose. One patient was given 300mcgs as a starting dose and told *"See how you get on."* The patient ended up in hospital badly overdosed.

12.   The same consultant had told her (before she was diagnosed with hypothyroidism) *"You are jealous of your teenage daughters and if you had a better social life and sex life then you would feel totally different."* Her thoughts were that she couldn't manage the life she had never mind another one.

13.   A patient had her thyroid function test returned "normal range" so the doctor said to her, *"How do you want to play it?"*

14.   Another patient had her thyroid function test returned 11.2. The scale used in her area is from 9.8 – 23. The doctor said, *"I can do nothing until you are outside the range."* The lady had many signs and symptoms.

15.   One lady pleaded with her doctor to help her and he just shouted. The patient cried all the way home.

The next seven quotations come through the helpline many times.

16.   *"Stop imagining you're ill."*
17.   *"Why should we give you something that is bad for you?"*
18.   *"Exercise more."*
19.   *"You are too placid for your own good."*
20.   *"You must be cheating on your diet to be so overweight."*
21.   *"I don't know what's the matter with you but I'll give you these antidepressants."*
22.   *"You are borderline but I can't give you any treatment until you go below the normal range."*

The next four quotations are utterly absurd:

23.   *"You will not grow hair under your arms because you are too fat."*
24.   *"You are not depressed because you are too fat. You are fat because you are depressed."*
25.   *"The doctor told me my loss of hearing was due to me being overweight."*
26.   *"Because you are single you don't have a normal life."* This was said to a female patient by a male consultant. Arrogant man!

Whatever happened to this doctor's initiative?

27.   *"You ought to have a thyroid problem but the blood test says you haven't."*

This one is amazing!

28.   One lady's eyebrows were very sparse. The G.P. said, *"You must have overplucked them in the 60's !!"*

Where is this one coming from?

29.   *"You can't treat people for a thyroid disorder just because they have the symptoms, because that would make a nonsense of science!"*

30. One G.P. said to a patient that the only way she would lose weight was if she fasted for two years, or go on a 500 calorie controlled diet. Both these statements are ludicrous and an insult to the patient whose self-esteem is already at a very low ebb.

31. Another patient was given two weeks supply of thyroxine and told she would feel fine. She was not told that she would have to be on the medication for life. She missed out on many months of treatment because she did not go back to the doctor straight away.

32. After being put on to treatment for an underactive thyroid gland, one lady lost a stone in two weeks. The G.P. panicked and took her off the treatment. She is getting steadily worse. Many patients lose a lot of weight once on thyroid replacement therapy. I did myself, 9 lbs to be exact. I call it the "thyroid weight".

33. One patient told her consultant she was going on holiday to Barbados. He immediately retorted, *"You shouldn't be going there you should be going skiing where you can cover up."*

34. A specialist told one lady that she was a *"chip and doughnut"* person and that she would have to stop eating those in order to lose weight.

35. Another lady was told, *"Go to bingo, at least you're not dead."*

36. G.P. to patient, *"The trouble is you can't cope with ageing."*

Consultant to patient:

37. *"Your thyroxine level is low but we can only rely on the blood tests."*

38. *"It's all in your head."*

These two quotations are outright rude.

123

39. *"Can't you just accept the fact that you are fat and losing hair?"*

40. One lady who was overweight was told, *"You mustn't be so vain, look at Rubens' women."*

I have saved the best quotation till last!

41. *"WE CAN'T GO BY WHAT YOU FEEL."*, quoted by three G.P.s to contacts on my helpline!

These quotations are just the tip of the iceberg, I have hundreds more.

For those G.P.s who say, "No fat people came out of Belsen," one could say that those people were not in Belson long enough to have the obesity connected with a low thyroid disorder! Many underactive thyroid sufferers are very, very, thin and look worn out.

There is only one thing that I can say about these quotations and that is that G.P.s and consultants have a very vivid imagination and maybe they would make better story-tellers.

You can get more respect out of a motor mechanic because he LISTENS TO THE ENGINE.

This chapter is not meant to condemn all doctors just to expose those who treat patients shabbily. Neither is it meant to condemn biochemists: only those who do not take into consideration the spectrum of factors which contribute to the regulation of thyroid metabolism.

G.P.s and consultants are taking symptoms out in isolation and treating them instead of looking at the whole picture. Because of this the patient suffers and is told, "You mustn't worry about the symptoms."

Unfortunately, many doctors are reacting badly to patients instead of responding to their needs and the patients then feel intimidated. They are told that they are imagining things and the reason why they went to the surgery in the first place has been forgotten and the patient then starts to mistrust their own perceptible abilities. This is not a happy relationship for either the patient or the doctor.

Once a doctor has that bit of paper in his hand, i.e. the thyroid blood test result, he or she relaxes, and if the blood test states normal, then the G.P. is happy. It would appear that the medical professional is now diagnosing blood tests instead of patients. There appears to be a role reversal, instead of patients telling the doctors how they feel, the doctor now tells the patient, "You're normal, there is nothing wrong with you."

When the blood test result had been returned to the doctor "within the normal range" he/she hangs on to that word "normal". He can't be sued if it states "normal". Doctors are afraid of litigation and who can blame them? In the main, this existing problem of misinterpretation of blood tests for thyroid function, has evolved with the passage of time.

Doctors have said to patients, "I can't give you something that is dangerous for you." Also, "It will weaken your heart muscles." Now we are talking about serious over-dosing here, when the patient becomes thyrotoxic (overactive). As long as the patient is put on to a very small dose of thyroxine and increases it very slowly and he/she is aware of the advantages and disadvantages then there should be no problem.

Patients who, for years, have been fit and well on their dosage of thyroxine, have their yearly blood test and are then told by their G.P. that he wishes to decrease their dose because they have become thyrotoxic as the result of the blood test is above the upper limit. The patients are never consulted as to whether or not they have thyrotoxic symptoms. The majority of these patients show no sign of overactivity. Their health then starts to decline.

Is it fair that patients should live a poor quality of life, sometimes for many years, just to fit in with a blood test result?

Now let us get one thing straight, you don't want to be in that surgery. In fact, before you decide to make the journey you debated with yourself whether or not you should attend for the appointment but you know that you are not well so you continue making trips to the surgery in case your G.P. finds the solution.

G.P.s are, of course, General Practitioners and are not supposed to be specialists in any one field.

Blood tests for thyroid function are carried out and when the result is returned in the "normal range", the G.P. then determines diagnosis and states the patient is "euthyroid" (euthyroid means the patient has normal thyroid function). "Normal range" does not necessarily mean the patient has "normal health" it merely means that the patient's level of hormone lies within the "normal range". Unfortunately, G.P.s are uneducated in this field.

A large majority of the contacts who rang me, after I featured in magazines, stated that they were never given a physical examination. In all the books I have read it states that for a suspected case of thyroid malfunction the doctor should take down signs, symptoms, history and carry out a clinical appraisal.

THIS IS NOT HAPPENING.

I say again that G.P.'s are not supposed to be specialists in every field but when something is brought to their notice they should at least take it on board.

The criteria are being met in part by the doctors and also by the laboratories but there is a missing link somewhere and therefore the patient misses out.

Now let us look at it from the point of view of the biochemists in the laboratory, the G.P,. the receptionist and the patient. You may indeed ask why the receptionist? All will be revealed.

BIOCHEMISTS: The biochemists understand how the reference ranges are made up and how to measure the hormone values in the blood, but neither see nor know the patient. How, then, can they interpret the blood test result?

126

G.P: The doctor knows the patient and the patient's signs and symptoms but does not know how the references ranges are arrived at.

RECEPTIONIST: The receptionist is given the responsibility of telling the patients the result of their blood test, and neither knows the patient nor how the reference values are made up.

PATIENTS: We are sometimes guilty of not taking enough evidence with us to the doctor's surgery. We tend to dwell on one or two symptoms instead of going prepared. Some patients have told me that their doctor is so nice that they do not want to upset him. NICE does not get you well.

So many times I have heard from patients that the G.P. tells them, "I can't give you thyroxine, it's bad for you."

Blood tests are always carried out for thyroid function before there is any thought of giving out medication. What about **H.R.T.** and **STEROIDS?** I was given **H.R.T.** and large doses of **STEROIDS** without having my hormone values checked. It would appear that there is one rule for one medication and a different rule for another.

There is something I would like to point out at this stage. A better check ought to be kept on patients' files at the G.P.'s surgery. Many patients, including myself, have found certain information missing. When the G.P.s are questioned about this they know nothing.

The next chapter will help you to prepare for your visit to the G.P.

CHAPTER TWELVE

HELP YOUR G.P. TO HELP YOU; TREATMENT; THE ROAD TO RECOVERY

Hypothyroidism comes in three stages:

> *1.* SUBCLINICAL *One or two symptoms that are not really troubling the patient - early stages.*
>
> *2.* CHRONIC *When the patient is grossly overweight with much swelling of the body and suffering from exhaustion and many more signs and symptoms or the patient looks older than their years and can be quite thin. Poor quality of life.*
>
> *3.* COMA *Death.*

Chronic hypothyroidism is so widespread and yet it is not picked up easily. There are three reasons why this could be happening.

The first reason for this is because the thyroid function tests are open to misinterpretation. The second reason is that chronic hypothyroidism is not being recognised. Thirdly, there are a wide range of presentations before the doctor and this confuses him.

The patient also is confused because one week one set of symptoms is to the fore and the next week it is another set of symptoms. This is truly happening to the patient. I know, I have been in that position. The doctor never writes down your signs and symptoms, he just takes in what you tell him on the day.

The first thing you can do is to list all your signs and symptoms.

Set out below is the complete list of signs and symptoms:

- Exhaustion, Lethargy, Sleepiness,
- Weight Gain, Puffiness (Eyes, Face, Hands, Feet Or Ankles) ,
- Muscle Or Joint Pain,
- Migraines, Headaches, Head Feels As If It Is Going To Explode ,
- Cramps, Lower Back Pain,
- Skin (Dry, Flaky, Coarse Patches)
- Complexion – Sallow (Yellowy) Pale, Flushed Or Normal.
- Brittle Nails, Flake Off, Soft,
- Hair Loss (Head, Pubic, Legs, Underarm, Eyebrows (Outer Edge),
- Intolerance To The Cold, Intolerance To Heat, Overheating, Breathlessness,
- Slow Movement, Slow Speech,
- Insomnia,
- Dizziness, Palpitations,
- Swallowing Difficulties, Lumpy Swallowing, Choking Fits Over Food Or Drink,
- Hoarse Voice, Dry Mouth, Tongue Feels Too Big For Your Mouth, Sore Throats,
- Carpal Tunnel Syndrome (Tendons Swell In The Wrist And Cause Numbness In The Hand Which Presses On Nerve Which Passes Through The Carpal Tunnel),
- Loss Of Sex Drive
- Numbness (Legs, Feet, Toes, Arms, Hands, Fingers, Back, Neck, Or Head),
- Visual Disturbances – Blurring, Poor Focusing, Double Vision,
- Light Sensitivity,

- Deafness, Noises In The Ears, Oversensitivity In Hearing,
- Constipation, Diarrhoea,
- Menstrual Disorders (Heavy Periods, Cessation Of Periods)
- Loss Of Appetite,
- Blood Pressure – High, Low Or Normal
- Sun-Sensitivity,
- Heavy Eyelids (Feel So Heavy That You Just Want To Go To Sleep),
- Palms Of The Hands (Red And Burn)
- Food Sensitivity, Alcohol Intolerance,
- Loss Of Balance, Feeling Disorientated,
- Pins And Needles,
- Panic Attacks,
- Memory Impaired, Concentration Poor,
- Cry Or Get Upset Easily, Mood Swings, Anger, Depression,
- Nervousness, Anxiety,
- Noises And Voices In The Head, Hallucinations, Claustrophobia, Any Other Phobias,
- Persecution Complex,
- Personality Change,
- Resentfulness Towards Partner, Family, Friends,
- Suspicious Of People's Motives,
- Lack Of Confidence,
- Wanting To Be On One's Own.

So now you have your list of signs and symptoms ready. Something else to have prepared is your medical history and family medical history so far as is known. For instance, are there any thyroid problems, heart problems, diabetes or any other major illnesses in the family?

Taking your basal temperature can tell you and your doctor what is happening at cell level. The Broda Barnes basal temperature method is the best.

STEP ONE: Upon retiring to bed leave a thermometer well shaken by the bedside.

STEP TWO: Before arising the next morning, place the thermometer under the armpit for ten minutes and then take a reading. If you can't get the hang of reading the thermometer ask the nurse at your G.P.'s surgery. Normal readings are between 97.8 – 98.4 degrees Fahrenheit and 36.6 – 37 degrees Celsius.

This simple test can show a malfunction at cell level, none of the sophisticated blood tests can do this.

There are those in the medical profession who say many other conditons give rise to a low basal temperature. These are, to say the least, very obvious conditions, i.e. alcoholism, hypothermia, surgical shock, hypoadrenalism, malnutrition, etc.

Next, if you do not already know how to take your pulse, then here is a step by step approach to taking your pulse.

Hold out your left hand and look to the base of the thumb. Follow the line outside of the wrist, for two inches. Then take the index finger and the middle finger of the right hand and half an inch in from the outer edge depress those two fingers (it's in the soft part). There you should feel your pulse. We have different rhythms so don't be afraid if yours is different from somebody else's. Take your pulse for one whole minute. This will give you a truer picture, some people take it for half a minute and then double it.

Normal pulse ranges are from 70 beats to 80 beats per minute with a margin of flexibility either side.

You are now prepared for your visit to the doctor. You have listed your signs and symptoms and written out, in brief, your clinical history. Take these, together with your pulse and temperature readings. If your doctor suspects a thyroid malfunction he should carry out a clinical appraisal and send a blood sample away to test for thyroid malfunction.

These are the ways in which you can help your doctor to help you, this is providing, of course, that your doctor plays his part. Too often however, I hear that the G.P. never carries out a clinical appraisal.

Here's hoping that your doctor will not let himself be tainted by apparent scepticism.

TREATMENT

Let us assume that the doctor has now decided upon a diagnosis of hypothyroidism (underactive thyroid). Your G.P. should start you on thyroxine. (T4) – a synthetic hormone. This is a replacement therapy. You will need to take this medication for the rest of your life, except in very rare cases.

CAUTION is the key word. If you have been ill for a number of years, or are over fifty years of age, then a starting dose of 25 micrograms is wise. The body needs time to adjust to a hormone that it has been deprived of for so long. If you are under fifty years of age and have had the condition for a few months then 50 micrograms may be in order.

Your medication should increase gradually over the months until you reach your optimum dose. This is the dose whereby you feel a sense of well-being. Many patients seem to go through a reversal of the illness before they get better.

Many G.P.s and consultants have given 100 micrograms to 300 micrograms as a starting dose with disastrous consequences, i.e. hospitalisation! Thyroxine is a powerful hormone and needs to be treated with respect and the patient must not be given too much too soon.

On the other hand, there are doctors out there who will not give thyroxine, even when there is overwhelming evidence that it is needed, stating that it is dangerous. This may relate back to the 30's when certain Harley Street doctors overdosed their patients on thyroid replacement therapy and then blamed the medication on the death of the patients.

OVERDOSING on any drug is potentially dangerous.

If you happen to go into an overdose situation then set out below is a list of signs and symptoms to watch for:

Many palpitations, rapid pulse, agitation, rapid weight loss, profuse sweating, restlessness, diarrhoea, nervousness, excitability and pain over the heart (angina pain) and hot sweats.

If you experience any of these signs or symptoms then return to your doctor immediately. He will most probably stop the medication for a few days until things have settled down and then start you off again until you reach the optimum dose with which you feel happy.

With the majority of patients once they have been diagnosed with an underactive thyroid the G.P. or consultant says, "Take these and you'll feel find." NO ADVICE – NO LITERATURE – NOTHING. The patient finds him/herself outside the surgery – with their mind in a whirl.

DON'T expect to get better in a few days – this will not happen – the body needs time to adjust to the medication. If you take your car to the garage for repair – remember it is not out on the road. It stays in the garage until it is in a road-worthy condition. In no way am I recommending that your body needs garaging – just to be patient. The thyroid is responsible for every single cell in the body, this means muscles, nerves, bones, etc., and it has a powerful influence on your well-being.

You may find that some signs and symptoms improve quite quickly whereas others may take up to twelve to eighteen months to clear or it can be as long as two-and-a-half years.

This is sometimes not easy. It can take many months to find the dose that is right for you.

Initially your G.P. will want to see you between six to eight week intervals. Once you have found your optimum dose then a yearly blood test for thyroid function is wise. If you have any real problems in the meantime then make an appointment with your G.P. as soon as possible.

After medication for an underactive thyroid has commenced you may experience some strange, odd or quirky feelings. Many of these are due to the fact that the body is undergoing repair work on a grand scale. Sometimes you may feel worse before you feel better. You may pass water a great deal – this is the body ridding itself, in the main, of mucopolysaccharides. This is good. The body makes mucopolysaccharides in normal quantities when the thyroid is functioning properly but mass produces them when the thyroid is under-functioning.

The following extract from Medicine International, 1993, is of interest:

> The aim of hypothyroidism is to normalize plasma TSH and to achieve a clinically euthyroid state. To obtain this, FT4 and TT4 have to be maintained at, or just above, the upper reference interval. In patients who have an abnormal TSH, either FT4 or TT4 levels must be measured to help to determine the required change in dose of thyroxine. Unless patients are seriously under treated or over treated, TT3 and FT3 are usually normal and T3 measurements are of little help in monitoring patients on TT4 replacement.
>
> Following a change in the prescribed dose of thyroxine, it may be many weeks before the thyroid function tests stabilize again. When the dose of thyroxine is increased, results do not stabilize for at least 6-8 weeks. If the dose of T4 is decreased, it may be

many months before normal thyrotroph responsiveness is restored; TSH results must therefore be interpreted with caution during this period.

DO'S AND DON'TS ON THE ROAD TO RECOVERY

- **DO NOT** OVER DO IT – if you do, you will suffer. Try and find a happy medium in everything you do whilst you are finding your optimum dose. Shortly after starting treatment you may be aware that your energy levels are raised and you begin to think clearly and you might think you are ready for anything. This is a mistake! Your body needs time to adjust. I remember only too well, once that first sense of well-being hit me, I thought I could take on the world. My body was not prepared for the onslaught and I paid dearly for being too foolish. I regressed badly, experiencing some of the same symptoms I had before treatment commenced.

- **Do not** expect everyone to come to terms with the "new you" straight away. They may need a time of adjustment. Those whose husbands, partners or carers have been looking after the 'fort' for a long time may feel hurt because you don't need them as much and may not be able to cope with the "new independent you". My husband, Norman, had to adjust, as he had fetched and carried for me for a long time, and when I made noises about wanting to be independent in some areas, he felt I no longer needed him. How wrong he was!

For years, I had lived a sheltered life away from dog-eat-dog type of people, and many times Norman was to waylay petty individuals who came along and tried to vilify the work that I was to become involved in.

I also needed to come to terms with feeling well.

- **DO NOT** take kelp alongside thyroid replacement therapy. Kelp tablets are derived from seaweed. Seaweed contains iodine. Too much iodine can induce

135

HYPERTHYROIDISM (overactive thyroid). Always take the advice of a qualified nutritionist or herbalist.

- **DO** monitor yourself when on thyroid replacement therapy. Heart patients monitor themselves and diabetics inject and monitor their insulin intake. By monitoring yourself, you can advise the doctor of any improvements or ill effects that have taken place.

- **DO** be patient – this is the key for a return to full health, especially if you have been ill for a long time. A gradual increase in medication is by far the best. If your medication is increased too soon you may experience symptoms not unlike an overactive thyroid.

- **DO** remember to remind your G.P. once you have determined your optimum dose, to do a blood test for thyroid function every twelve months.

- **DO** listen to your body. It is a very good thing to be observant about our bodies. For instance, when we eat something that we know disagrees with us, why do we carry on?

WHEN A PATIENT IS ON
THYROID REPLACEMENT THERAPY
PRESCRIPTIONS ARE FREE.

Natural desiccated thyroid is an alternative replacement therapy and notably the brand "Armour" thyroid is excellent. Unfortunately, it is no longer in the British National Formulary. Many years ago, all desiccated thyroid was removed from the British National Formulary because with some brands there was a variation in strength with each tablet. There is no variation in strength with "Armour" thyroid. Desiccated thyroid is obtained from, in the main, pigs liver and has both hormones T4 and T3 and perhaps factor X.

I, myself, take "Armour" thyroid and have that extra "feel good" factor.

136

Many doctors are now starting to prescribe desiccated thyroid again. If you feel that you would like to try "Armour" thyroid then talk to your G.P.

Looking back, I have so much to thank God for. I try to do this each day and spend a quiet time with him in prayer and reading my Bible.

CHAPTER THIRTEEN

THE ENDOCRINE SYSTEM

The endocrine system is a group of glands in the body which manufacture hormones daily. This is necessary for the physical and mental well-being of the body. If these hormones are out of balance, then many areas of the body will be affected as they all interact with each other.
The endocrine system comprises:

HYPOTHALAMUS: The hypothalamus in the brain releases a hormone called thyrotrophin-releasing hormone. (known as T.R.H.) which in turn stimulates the pituitary to produce thyroid stimulating hormone.

PITUITARY: The pituitary gland lies at the base of the skull and is about the size of a little finger nail. It secretes various hormones for growth and also stimulating hormones for the thyroid, adrenal cortex and the ovaries in the female and testes in the male.

THYROID: The thyroid is responsible for the energy transformation in every single cell in your body. Another way of putting it – the thyroid is responsible for the metabolism in every single cell in your body.
The thyroid gland lies at the front of the neck. It is butterfly in shape and each wing sits on either side of the Adam's apple. The thyroid gland makes hormones for distribution round the body. The hormones are thyroxine (known as T4) and tri-iodothyronine (known as T3) and also calcitonin.
A small amount of T3 and a larger amount of T4 is produced. T3 is the more active hormone. T4 is converted to T3. T3 is active at cell level. There is a feed-back

mechanism to the pituitary. If the thyroid is failing to produce enough hormones, the pituitary sends a T.S.H. (thyroid stimulating hormone) to induce the thyroid to make more hormone.

CALCITONIN: regulates the amount of calcium taken from the bones into the plasma.

PANCREAS: supplies the duodenum with digestive fluid and secretes insulin into the blood.

ADRENALS: We each have two adrenal glands that are close to the top of the kidneys. An adrenal gland is made up of two parts. The first part is the inner, called the medulla which produces the stress hormones such as adrenaline and noradrenaline. These regulate heart beat and blood pressure. The second part is the outer called the cortex. This produces steroids such as hydrocortisone. These hormones help convert carbohydrate into energy. They are also responsible for the sex hormones such as oestrogen, progesterone and testosterone. Under-productivity by the adrenal glands can bring on **Addison's** disease.

Signs and symptoms of Addison's disease are weight loss, malaise, weakness, nausea, gastro-intestinal problems, diarrhoea or constipation, postural hypotension (this is when you get up from a lying down position and your blood pressure falls), brown pigmentation, decreased body hair - especially in the female.

Over-productivity by the adrenal glands can bring on **Cushing's** disease.

Signs and symptoms of Cushing's disease are weight gain, hirsutism (excessive growth of hair on the face or body), backache, muscle weakness, moonface, hypertension, bruising, striae (bluish stretch marks on the tummy).

GONADS: Ovaries in female and Testes in male. These organs are responsible for reproduction.

139

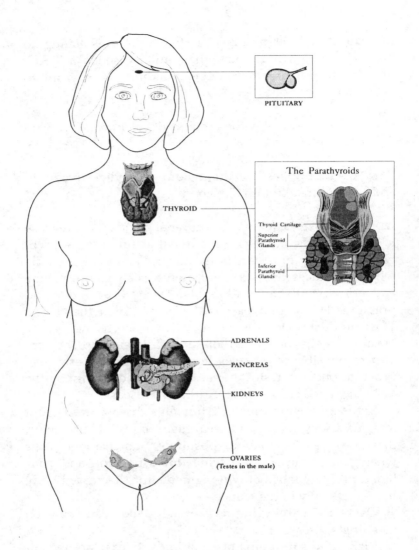

PITUITARY

THYROID

The Parathyroids

Thyroid Cartilage

Superior
Parathyroid
Glands

Inferior
Parathyroid
Glands

ADRENALS

PANCREAS

KIDNEYS

OVARIES
(Testes in the male)

**DIAGRAM SHOWING THE KEY COMPONENTS OF
THE ENDOCRINE SYSTEM.**

N.B. The kidneys are <u>not</u> part of the endocrine system but are shown here so
as to give a clear idea of where the adrenals are situated.

140

CHAPTER FOURTEEN

CONCLUSION

Chronic hypothyroidism is a common diagnostic failure.

It is sometimes called "mild myxoedema" but to those who suffer it is certainly not mild.

Laboratories are working on the assumption, for blood testing for thyroid function, that there is "an assumed fixed basis of comparison of so-called healthy people", so-called being the operative word. When the starting point is very loose then the end result cannot be deemed to be specific! The patients did not have a blood test when they were well, there was no need, so the doctor does not have a base-line from which to work.

The majority of G.P.'s and consultants do not know how the reference values are made up. Results are interpreted without any flexibility and therefore there is a problem with the diagnosis and management of hypothyroidism.

The patient has a poor quality of life through ill-health, sometimes for many many years. **This leads to lost potential.**

Continued ill-health that mystifies doctors in turn incurs exaggerated costs for the N.H.S. for each patient.

Let us hypothesise. Assuming that there are thousands and thousands of missed cases of hypothyroidism and thousands and thousands of diagnosed treated cases still not well out there, then what illnesses have they been diagnosed with? How many, laparoscopy, tonsillectomy and hysterectomy operations have been performed when there was no need?

I would like to recap on the mis-diagnoses that were given me, bearing in mind that I wasn't suffering from any of these illnesses but from hypothyroidism and hypoadrenalism.

141

Epilepsy: *Hypothyroidism can manifest symptoms of epilepsy.*

Coeliac disease: *In hypothyroidism there are problems throughout the digestive system.*

Polmyalgia rheumatica: *muscle weakness is apparent in hypothyroidism.*

Depression: *is a known symptom of hypothyroidism.*

M.E.: *manifests all the signs and symptoms of hypothyroidism.*

Myasthenia gravis: *the neuro transmitters are faulty. I had a tensilon test which proved positive. I do not suffer with myasthenia gravis. How many more people have been diagnosed with this disease, under such a test and the test has proved positive yet in reality they do not have the disease? The tensilon test cannot be deemed to be the determining factor for diagnosis in myasthenia gravis. This is an area that needs much more research.*

Out of the six diseases listed, a percentage of patients, who have been diagnosed with any of them, might be suffering from hypothyroidism.

Low thyroid function brings about a deposition of mucopolysaccharides and Dr. Broda Barnes believed that this was the possible cause of degenerative diseases such as heart related conditions:

Atherosclerosis: furring up of the arteries.

Hypercholesterolemia: high cholesterol levels.

Hypertension:: high blood pressure.

Angina pectoris: an attack of intense restricting pain in the chest, brought on by exertion, due to an inadequate blood supply to the heart.

It is a known fact that atherosclerosis and hypercholesterolemia can cause heart attacks and hypertension can cause strokes.

There are many other diseases into which the missed cases of hypothyroidism can be pigeon-holed.

The diagnosed treated cases not on enough treatment will gradually become worse.

DIABETES: It is possible for a low functioning thyroid to cause diabetic complications. Thyroid therapy could prevent the vascular complications.

SCHIZOPHRENIA: Many of the symptoms of schizophrenia can also be symptomatic of hypothyroidism. I myself had noises and voices in the head, voices which told me to do dreadful things. Also hallucinations, these are typical symptoms of schizophrenia. Since a diagnosis of hypothyroidism and subsequent treatment I have none of those symptoms. There could be a percentage in this schizophrenic group that have been mis-diagnosed.

DEPRESSION: If we were to take notice of the medical profession on this one then practically the whole of the women in the U.K. would be suffering from what is known as "clinical depression". I am not and would never advocate that all depressed people are suffering from a low thyroid disorder.

There are, of course, many depressive illnesses. Hypothyroidism has its own depression brought about by the illness. It is not being recognised. The G.P. or consultant, takes depression from a long list of signs and symptoms and treats it, to the exclusion of every other symptom that the patient is experiencing. It would appear that the medical profession is taking out symptoms, in isolation, and treating them all singularly instead of looking at all of the patient's symptoms.

Doctors glibly diagnose depression today time after time, not seeing it sometimes for the symptom it can be as part of a very complex physiological problem. I am, of course, referring to hypothyroidism or hyperthyroidism.

POST-NATAL DEPRESSION: It is known that when a woman is pregnant her thyroid hormone levels go up and come down after lactation. If twelve months after the birth of her baby the mother is still feeling depressed, with accompanying symptoms, then a thyroid function test is wise. Depression is most often treated solely with antidepressants.

OBESITY: Many patients with hypothyroidism have a weight problem. No amount of dieting can shift the weight. Some of it is mucopolysaccharides, some water retention and some fat weight that will not burn off because the metabolism is too sluggish. The mucopolysaccharides and water retention are lost fairly quickly once medication is started and you may find that you have lost quite a few pounds without even trying Once you are well, the rest of your surplus weight may be lost on a controlled diet with Weight Management or a similar slimming club.

However, many hypothyroid sufferers do not lose the weight that they expect to once on thyroid replacement therapy. More research is needed in this area.

Mucopolysaccharides are made by the body normally but when the thyroid is underactive they mass produce and infiltrate all over the body. This accounts for most of the puffiness in hypothyroidism.

MIGRAINE/HEADACHE: Migraine and headaches are very common in hypothyroid sufferers.

LUPUS: This is a connective tissue disorder. Mucopolysaccharides infiltrate into all connective tissue in hypothyroidism.

ARTHRITIS & RHEUMATISM: Rheumatoid and arthritic aches and pains, sometimes of great severity, are experienced by patients with low thyroid disorder.

BREATHLESSNESS: This is sometimes confused with asthma and again people are put on to medication for the symptom and diagnosed as asthmatic, when many many more signs and symptoms that the patient suffers from should be taken into account. Many patients with a low functioning thyroid suffer breathlessness.

MENSTRUAL DISORDERS: Heavy periods and cessation of periods are typical symptoms of low thyroid disorder.

The output of thyroid hormone during menses is low and women start to experience the classic symptoms of hypothyroidism i.e. headaches, migraines, lower back pain, weariness and constipation.

Only when the period has ended do the levels rise again. But when the period is exceptionally heavy then that is the time to look to the thyroid and possible replacement therapy. Many a hysterectomy could have been prevented if this code of practice had been followed. According to a Belgian doctor, Eugene Hertoghe, in 1914, the weaker the thyroid the greater the loss of blood.

How many women have been curetted (D&C) unnecessarily?

INFERTILITY: People with low thyroid function are often infertile.

Dr. Eugene Hertoghe stated, in 1914, that thyroid replacement therapy had proved in scores of cases an excellent remedy for otherwise inexplicable sterility.

> *There are many more diseases that could be affected by low thyroid output.*

SKIN DISORDERS: Some forms of excema, psoriasis and alopecia can be caused by an underactive thyroid, as can vitiligo.

DIGESTIVE DISORDERS: Numerous digestive disorders can be related to a thyroid disorder. The intestinal secretion is inadequate, the walls of the bowels become lazy giving rise to constipation. The pancreatic juices are not the same and subsequently, the patient suffers from chronic indigestion.

DEMENTIA AND ALZHEIMER'S DISEASE: Some of the symptoms of these diseases are seen in hypothyroid cases. Care should be taken not to label a patient unless everything has been taken into consideration re hypothyroidism. I cannot stress enough that a doctor takes into account signs, symptoms and history and carries out a clinical appraisal using the blood test as an indicator only. It would appear that many times the doctor has no interest in the patient's signs and symptoms, in fact, even dismisses them.

CHRONIC MALNUTRITION & ALCOHOLISM: These conditions cause a shock to the thyroid gland and has an effect on the hormonal output.

SHOCK: Any kind of shock can trigger hypothyroidism such as: surgery, birth, bereavement, accident, overdosing on medication or undue stress over a long period.
Shock from chemo-therapies and high doses of steroids and radium treatment. Should the thyroid be checked when these treatments are given?

VIETNAM AND FALKLANDS WAR VETERANS

These men have undergone shock and undue stress over a long period. Should the thyroid be checked?

If G.P.s and consultants could give more clinical evidence when requesting a blood test for thyroid function this may indeed help the laboratory technicians.
I think that the relationship between the laboratory experts and practitioners must be redefined, whereby there is much more communication and new guidelines need to be set. Doctors must reappraise their knowledge of

147

hypothyroidism if they are to be responsible for diagnosing and managing this condition.

The medical world has become too cautious about the diagnosis of hypothyroidism. This may stem back to the 1930's when certain doctors gave thyroid replacement therapy in large doses. The heart would then race beyond its capability and this brought on heart attacks and in some instances, death. This flagrant mis-use gave thyroid replacement therapy a bad name. Subsequently, doctors are now erring on the side of over-caution, so much so that, in some cases, patients who have been on medication for as long as twenty years and have felt very well, have had their medication decreased because the blood test result was returned "normal". Their health is in decline but the G.P.'s are adamant that they are treating the patient correctly.

Rigidity with the interpretation of blood tests for thyroid function is causing people to be ill longer than is necessary and subsequently their adrenal glands can become exhausted. This is yet another problem that is not being recognised..

The Royal College of General Practitioners maintains, "It is crucial that the doctor treats the patient and not the blood test result." There has been failure to observe this resulting in many women being told that, as the blood test result was within the "normal range", no treatment is required. Clinically, the woman is no better. In addition, she is told she has a psychosomatic disorder typical of a woman compounded by the fact that her doctor declares, "We can't go by what you feel."

Thyroid conditions mainly seem to affect women. Although I believe there may be more men suffering with the complaint than is yet known. There are complex issues that could be involved here.

WOMEN: Women suffer more physically than men in many ways, for example, we go through the menses, give birth, and may have gynaecological operations and finally

148

end up with the menopause. We appear to manifest more symptoms than men or is it just that we talk about them more?

Secondly, many woman are doing twice as much as they used to in as much as they are looking after the children, running a home and working full-time. All this adds up to stress. Stress affects the thyroid.

MEN: Why don't men appear to suffer with these conditions as much as women? Maybe it's just that it is not macho to complain about symptoms and so they suffer. All this is, of course, conjecture but to any man reading this book, it is all right to complain of symptoms no matter how insignificant they seem to you.

OTHER REASONS WHY THERE IS A PREPONDERANCE OF HYPOTHYROIDISM TODAY

- The air we breath is contaminated by fumes and chemical pollutants.
- The water we drink has added chemicals that are known to be bad for the thyroid, i.e. fluoride and chlorine.
- The food we eat has been sprayed with pesticides (containing organo phosphates) and injected with hormones, i.e. oestrogen and antibiotics.
- The pace of life today is fast and although our brains are trying to cope our bodies still haven't caught up yet. It takes many many years for the body to evolve.
- Thyroid conditions are most definitely in the ante-social diseases category. Most people suffering want to shut themselves away.

PERSONAL RELATIONSHIPS

This is one area that is very difficult. The sufferers are having a hard time coping with their own bodies never mind what is going on in the home regarding relationships. The patient knows he/she is not well, sometimes the partner or carer think that the patient is putting on an act. Other carers feel for the sufferer because they are so helpless.

Nevertheless this brings about unhappy relationships whichever way you look at it. The majority of patients suffer with anger, mood swings, depression and resentfulness. If you put that ingredient into a family relationship trouble is bound to ensue. How many marriages have failed or relationships suffered because of the misinterpretation of thyroid tests?

The patient has been to the doctor so many times with the result that the G.P. says that there is nothing wrong with them. This naturally upsets the patient but the partner or carer begins to think that they may be making it up – is it all an act?

The strength for patients to stand up for themselves is conspicuous by its absence.

The partner or carer because of the unhappy situation at home takes his grievances or his concerns into the work place which in turn affects his performance.

For those patients who are missed cases of hypothyroidism and for the diagnosed treated cases of hypothyroidism who are still not well and are mismanaged, the work place can be a nightmare. You know that you are not as efficient as you should be but just let anyone tell you that. Every day you crawl into work and do your best.

The missed diagnoses and insufficiently treated cases of hypothyroidism and hyperthyroidism could be causing a great problem of inefficiency that is in the work place today, from both sufferers and the carers.

WHY ADDRESSING THE PROBLEM OF DIAGNOSING HYPOTHYROIDISM IS OF SUCH GREAT IMPORTANCE.

All People who are suffering from hypothyroidism are affected by all sorts of maladies as set out below:

ADULTS:

- Stubborn obesity,
- exhaustion,
- lack of motivation,
- depression,
- mood disturbances,
- progressive failure of memory and concentration,
- skin and hair problems,
- rheumatic illness,
- migraines and headaches,
- digestive disorders and constipation,
- menstrual disorders,
- infertility.

CHILDREN:

(NB: In a paper sent to us on hypothyroidism (Broda O. Barnes MD and Lawrence Galton (1976): 'The Unsuspected Illness', New York, Thomas Y. Cromwell) it says that a few children suffering from hypothyroidism will be very nervous, hyperactive and unusually aggressive. Emotional problems are frequent. A low thyroid child may cry for no apparent reason, and object vigorously to any restrictions. Temper tantrums are common, probably related to undue fatigue. The child may sleep for longer than other youngsters of his or her age, be a slow starter in the mornings and have a short attention span and flit from one activity to another and infections are common. We can recall one child who was so diagnosed by her homeopathic doctor and made a really good recovery after treatment. If you think your child shows the sort of symptoms mentioned, it might be worth seeking advice, perhaps through a homeopathic doctor (always shown in the local telephone book).

- Behavioural disorders leading to total exclusion from school,
- poor growth, intelligence and learning,
- chronic illness,
- catarrhal child syndrome,
- poor sleep and appetite.

THE ELDERLY: (although all adults can be affected in the same way)

151

- atherosclerosis - leading to heart disease,
- hypercholesterolemia - high cholesterol levels,
- hypothermia,
- increased susceptibility to illness,
- causes complications in diabetes,
- respiratory illness.

All this, of course, adds to the National Health Service costs, which leads me nicely into expenditure.

EXPENDITURE:

The amount of money I alone spent was in the thousands and since being involved with the helpline so many people have told me of the vast amounts of money that they have spent in trying to regain their health. This of course, is draining their private funds unnecessarily.

Here is a list of mainstream and alternative medicines that patients have tried in order regain their health.

There is no order of preference.

Mainstream:
- Endocrinologist (deals with thyroid and other parts of the endocrine system),
- Rheumatologist,
- Gynaecologist,
- Gastroenterologist,
- Orthodontist,
- Psychiatrist,
- Dermatologist,
- Physiotherapist,
- Menopause clinic.

ALTERNATIVE MEDICINES:
- Homeopathy,
- Osteopathy,
- Acupuncture (I have had some very good results from acupuncture)
- Hydrotherapy,
- Chiropractice,

- Reflexology (I personally have great faith in reflexologists. They can pin-point where in the body it is diseased).
- Iridology,
- Kniesiology,
- Faith-healing,
- Aromatherapy (This can be a very soothing treatment),
- Nutritionists, (Consulting one can put you in the right direction regarding vitamins and minerals that your body requires.)

All these are tried with little or no improvement in many cases.

NATIONAL HEALTH SERVICE FUNDING.

Each missed case of hypothyroidism and diagnosed treated cases still not well has had a vast amount of money spent on them by the N.H.S. Whether it be blood tests, x-rays, physiotherapy, operations, referral to consultants, medication (i.e. antidepressants) etc., all of which may have been unnecessary.

Much more clarity is needed together with a consensus of opinion within the medical world on diagnosing and managing thyroid disorders.

It was once stated that, "progress in medicine is sometimes halted through mans' arrogance. It is only pure persistence that wins through."

We are certainly not progressing. **We are going backwards.**

As a former sufferer, I have great empathy with those who suffer, yet also feel for the G.P.s nowadays. They are expected to be high-powered administrators. They have a meagre five to eight minutes with each patient and are expected to diagnose them in this time. They must feel frustrated when they believe that they have correctly diagnosed a patient only to be dictated to by a blood test result.

G.P.s are given the responsibility of diagnosing and managing thyroid conditions that they know relatively little about. **Is this really fair to them?**

But G.P.s are not entirely blameless. How many patients today have had a clinical appraisal from their G.P. (full physical examination)? Does he write down all your signs and symptoms – no, because he has come to rely on the blood tests. They were never ever meant to be the sole determining factor for diagnosis.

We are not entirely blameless either. Doctors today, are afraid of litigation – afraid of being sued so they opt for the safe way out – the blood test result reads in the "normal range" but does not read that the patient is in "normal" health.

The time has come for new guidelines to be set for doctors diagnosing and managing thyroid conditions.

Dr. Broda Barnes once stated:

> *"Have we arrived at a super scientific endeavour, in which the way a patient feels plays no role in his treatment and must he modify himself to fit the errors of a machine? GOD FORBID!"*

I personally believe the misinterpretation of thyroid function tests to be the biggest *faux pas* in medical history. **Medicine is not an exact science and it never will be.**

This concludes my studies to date and I have made recommendations to the Department of Health set out as follows:

RECOMMENDATIONS

1. A change in clinical practice regarding the interpretation of thyroid function tests. Results of thyroid function tests not to be the sole determining factor for diagnosis and that signs and symptoms and

patients history are taken into account and a clinical appraisal carried out.

2. Doctors to re-appraise their knowledge of thyroid conditions. Much more clarity together with a consensus of opinion, within the medical profession, on diagnosis and management of thyroid disorders.
3. Nurses to counsel newly diagnosed thyroid sufferers.
4. Literature re thyroid conditions to be made readily available at the G.P.'s surgery.
5. If patients, who believe that they have a thyroid condition and would like to take some responsibility for their own health and wish to try a trial of thyroxine, they should be given the option of a disclaimer, provided that both the advantages and disadvantages of the therapy are explained, then neither the doctor nor patient would be disadvantaged.
6. Everyone from the age of twenty one should have a thyroid function test carried out. This will determine the base-line for each person.
7. Thyroid medication alone to be free on prescription and not all other medication.

IMPORTANT: If you agree in principle with the 7 recommendations set out above then please write to me stating this to be so. Each letter will form part of the Patient Empowerment Plan that is to be put forward.

Write to:

Diana Holmes,
c/o The Community Health Council,
45 Queen Street,
Wolverhampton,
West Midlands,
WV1 3BJ

God bless you!
Diana Holmes

155

- **In 1877,** Dr. William Ord, a brilliant London physician, performed a post-mortem examination of a mature woman. Her thyroid gland was so overgrown and choked with fibrous tissue that it had stopped functioning and she showed advanced signs of atherosclerosis. He named the condition "myxoedema" ("myx" meaning mucin and "oedema" meaning swelling).
- **In 1890,** Viennese pathologists discovered thryroid deficiency brings on heart attacks.
- **In 1944,** Dr. Zondek wrote *Discoveries of the Endocrine Gland* which was translated into English in 1944. He noted that the E.C.G.s of some patients showed low voltage because of weak heart beats. After thyroid therapy E.C.G.s returned to normal.

When the National Health Service was formed fifty years ago, it was hoped that spending would rise sharply then fall. The assumption was that chronic illness would be stamped out at an early stage, and the N.H.S. would gradually produce a healthier society.

This has not happened. We have spent billions of pounds trying to make poorly people better but treating symptoms instead of getting to the root of the problem. The N.H.S. never stood a chance.

Around the same time that the N.H.S. came into being, drugs were being used to combat T.B. and so patients were cured of this disease and lived beyond the age whereby T.B would have killed them.

Although these patients were living longer, they were now open to other diseases which could kill them, such as heart disease, diabetic complications, atherosclerosis, hypoglycemia, hypertension, hypercholesterolemia, hypothyroidism, etc.

156

APPENDIX I

CORRESPONDENCE

Letter from World Health Organisation, dated 26 July, 1994

Dear Mrs Holmes,

Your letter of 15 July 1994 to WHO was given to me for reply. I read your comments on "The reliability of blood tests for hypothyroidism" with great interest. Although I am not a specialist in hormone investigations, and particularly in the analysis of thyroid hormones or relating factors, I understand that the problem you address is valid for any laboratory test, and most professionals working in the laboratory are aware of the limits of interpretation of laboratory results and particularly of border line cases. You rightly say that the "normal" range may not be an appropriate reference for decision making. Indeed this is why laboratory experts are recommending to abandon the term "normal range" and replace it by "reference interval", while keeping in mind that the limit values for the reference interval will depend on the selected population that was investigated for their establishment.

On the other hand it is also clear from the ways of establishing such limits that they are the result of a statistical analysis and therefore are prone to some degree of uncertainty, which again will depend on the design of the investigations.

Finally, experts in laboratory diagnosis of thyroid disease do not stop to point out that in individual cases the levels of thyroid hormones may well be within the so called normal range in patients with thyroid disease, and the existing disease can only be diagnosed properly by investigating the spectrum of factors contributing to the regulation of thyroid metabolism.

It should also be emphasised that there are considerable differences in results of measurements for technical reasons, and this is particularly true in hormone measurement. No doubt that the clinician must be aware of all the limitations when taking care for a patient on the basis of laboratory investigations only.

157

Unfortunately we often observe an unsatisfactory communication between the laboratory and the practitioners, which may in some cases be the reason for misinterpretation of laboratory results.

I very much appreciate your efforts in drawing attention to this problem.

Best wishes,

Yours sincerely,

Dr. C.C. Heuck,

Health Laboratory Technology and Blood Safety

Letter from Department of Health dated 4th April, 1995.

Dear Mrs Holmes

Thank you and your colleagues very much for coming to the Department to discuss hypothyroidism on 14th March. I said I would record in summary form the nature of our discussions and send you some references. Thank you for your letter of 20th March and the enclosed references.

You and your colleagues describe two types of patient with hypothyroidism and from the numbers of letters you have received both types seem to be commonplace. In the first type a person is diagnosed as having hypothyroidism, is treated with thyroxine and their thyroid function tests return to the normal range. The person is not given the opportunity to see if a further increase in dose makes them feel better still or actually makes them worse because they become hyperthyroid. In the second type the person has the symptoms of hypothyroidism and normal thyroid function tests; the diagnosis of hypothyroidism is then dismissed and the person is labelled with a number of other diagnoses, most commonly depression.

I said that I think there are two reasons why there is a medico-scientific problem. The first is that the normal range of thyroid function tests is based on the measurements from a healthy population; by definition, 2% of the healthy population have measurements below the normal range and 2% of the healthy population have measurements above the normal range. Thus 2% are, by definition, hypothyroid. The second problem relates to the intra-individual day-to-day variability in thyroid function tests. The normal range for TSH, for instance, is roughly 0.5 to 5 mU per mL. A change of greater than .08 mU per mL in an

158

individual's measurement, assuming no intercurrent illness, is a significant change. Consequently, a person having a TSH of 1.5 on one occasion and subsequently a TSH of 3.5 has had a significant rise in his/her TSH, yet both are within the normal range. I said that were a person "lucky" enough to have such repeat measurements of thyroid function tests, most physicians would say "we have now had two tests of your thyroid function and both of them show that your thyroid is working normally".

I suggested that there were two ways of handling the issue of day-to-day variability in thyroid function tests; one is to stimulate some research and the other is to make patients with treated hypothyroidism aware that they may benefit from a further increase in their thyroxine therapy even if their thyroid function tests are within the normal range. A relatively easy research study to conduct is to take a group of patients with treated hypothyroidism with thyroid function tests within the normal range and randomise them for several weeks to receive twice their present dose of thyroxine, their present dose of thyroxine,or half their present dose of thyroxine (each person taking the same number of tablets using placebo tablets as necessary). A number of outcome measure such as the SF36 or the general health questionnaire before and after the change in treatment could be used. I made no commitment that the Department would fund research in this area.

Thank you again for the interesting discussion.

Yours sincerely,

Peter Bourdillon

Head of Specialist Clinical Services Division.

Letter from the Royal College of General Practitioners dated 23 October 1995.

Dear Mrs Holmes,

Thank you for your letter of 23 August 1995 regarding thyroid function tests. My apologies if it seems to have taken some time to reply to your letter, but I was keen to consult with colleagues to ensure a broad consensus of opinion before replying to your letter.

You do indeed highlight a problem that we have with many tests in that the reference ranges, by definition, include only ninety-five percent of normal people. With respect to thyroid function tests, however, this problem should be less important because it is a disease where it is crucial that the doctor treats the patient and not the blood test result.

For patients who are diagnosed as hypothyroid, whose blood test returns to within the reference range but is still unwell, then it would be very reasonable to treat that patient with Thyroxine. For those patients who appear to suffer from hypothyroidism but whose blood result is within the reference range, then the general practitioner appears to have two options. One is to try a small dose of Thyroxine to see if the patient clinically improves or, secondly, to refer the patient for a specialist opinion. Whatever action the GP takes, if the patient remains unwell, it would not seem unreasonable for the patient to be referred, even if the GP considers that he has excluded hypothyroidism as a diagnosis.

There is a theoretical drawback with treating patients with presumed thyroid deficiency, in this way – and that is where the diagnosis is not supported by blood tests: it is that the doctor may cause an illness through medication. Provided both the advantages and disadvantages are explained to patients so that they can make an informed decision, together with their GP, then it seems unlikely that either patient or their general practitioners would be disadvantaged.

I will agree with your suggestion that further research in this area would be helpful. It is also important for general practitioners to be mindful that a small percentage of normal patients will fall out with the reference range – and similarly, there will be a few abnormal patients who fall within them.

Yours sincerely,

Dr Bill Reith

Honorary Secretary of Council

Letter from Committee on Safety of Medicines dated 4th January 1996.

Dear Mrs Holmes

Thank you for your letter of 27 November 1995 to the Committee on Safety of Medicines regarding your concerns over thyroxine usage in hypothyroidism. I have been asked to reply on their behalf. Please accept my apologises for the delay in replying to your letter.

The general consensus of the medical profession is that in hypothyroidism the initial adult dosage of thyroxine should be 50 to 100 mcg daily, increased by increments of 25 to 50mcg at intervals of 3-4 weeks, until the thyroid deficiency is corrected and a maintenance dose has been established. The adult maintenance dose is usually between 100 to 200mcg daily. In older patients (over 50 years of age), in those with cardiac insufficiency, or in those with severe long-standing hypothyroidism, treatment should be introduced more gradually using lower initial doses, smaller increments and longer intervals between increases as necessary. An initial dose of 25mcg daily increased by increments of 25mcg at intervals of 4 weeks may be appropriate in such cases. In children, individualisation of doses and monitoring of treatment is especially important. In infants a daily dose of 10mcg/kg up to a maximum of 50mcg daily should be given. Subsequent therapy should reach 100mcg by 5 years and 100mcg to 20mcg by 12 years, guided by clinical response, growth assessment and measurement of plasma thyroxine and thyroid-stimulating hormone.

If the above guidelines are followed, these dosage regimes should be satisfactory for the majority of patients. Adverse effects of thyroxine are generally due to too rapid and/or too high doses, with symptoms which may include tachycardia, palpitations, anginal pain, headaches, nervousness and excitability. These adverse reactions normally disappear after dosage reduction or temporary withdrawal of treatment.

As I am sure you will appreciate, I cannot comment on the treatment of individual patients. The prescribing of medicines is for the clinical judgement of the doctor who is responsible for the treatment and who is familiar with the clinical history of the patient.

I hope this if some help to you.

Yours sincerely,

Dr. Tharani Sivananthan,

Scientific Assessor

Pharmacovigilance Assessment Group

APPENDIX II

AN ARTICLE BY ALISON WICK, *DAILY TELEGRAPH*, HEALTHFRONT, SATURDAY OCTOBER 11, 1997

THYROID DIAGNOSIS:
Some doctors now believe that tests do not tell the whole story.

Diana Holmes' first symptoms – dizziness and exhaustion – started in her late 20's. Then she started having fainting spells and was told she had epilepsy. Bowel problems led to a specialist diagnosing coeliac disease – an allergy to gluten – and she spent 11 years on a restricted diet. Severe muscle pain led to a diagnosis of polymyalgia rheumatica, a muscle disease, and she was sent to psychiatrists for depression. Other conditions she has been told she had are myalgic encephalomyelitis (ME) and myasthenia gravis, a serious neuromuscular disease.

Mrs Holmes, 54, a housewife and mother-of three from Wolverhampton put on two stone and even spent time in a wheelchair, too weak to move. But her nightmare ended three years ago.

'I went to see a private doctor and he suspected that I had a thyroid problem just by looking at me. I'd had at least one thyroid function test in the past but was told my thyroid was normal,' explains Mrs Holmes.

She was give a trial of thyroxine hormone and her recovery was dramatic. 'I got well and then wanted to know why. It made me angry that such an easy treatment could make me better and I wanted to know why the thyroid function tests could show I was in the normal range, and why my symptoms had been ignored.'

162

The thyroid gland, the size of a plum and lying across the windpipe in the throat, is responsible for many body processes, but its mains job is to control metabolism in the body's cells. If the gland produces too little thyroxine, the system slows down. Typically, patients complain of exhaustion, feeling cold, miserable and lethargic, weight gain, a husky low-pitched voice and menstrual disturbances – in fact, many wide-ranging symptoms.

Some would say Mrs Holmes is now on a crusade. She has taken her story to magazines and regional newspapers and has had a huge response on the telephone help-line from women who have suffered similar experiences. She has contacted endocrinologists (hormone specialists) and medical organisations to stop what she sees as an over-reliance on chemical tests while ignoring physical symptoms,

It seems strange that the controversy has even arisen, considering hypothyroidism is so common. 'It occurs in around seven per cent of women in the UK who are aged 45 or over,' says Sir Richard Bayliss, a consultant endocrinologist at the Lister Hospital, London.

There are two blood tests frequently used to assess thyroid function. One measures thyroxine and the other TSH (thyroid stimulating hormone), which is secreted from the pituitary gland to stimulate the thyroid gland. If TSH levels are abnormally high, this suggests insufficient thyroxine is being produced.

Sir Richard agrees that in the early stages of the disease, thyroxine levels may be normal with TSH just slightly raised – leading to some patients not being treated. 'There is no doubt from my clinical experience, that some of these people do get symptoms and their symptoms respond to thyroxine.' he says. The question now arising whether those with normal TSH levels should get treatment, too.

Rather than relying less on blood results, Sir Richard believes doctors should do more intensive investigations when the diagnosis is uncertain – such as looking for thyroid antibodies, which can indicate an autoimmune condition called Hashimoto's disease – the most common cause of thyroid deficiency.

One of the difficulties of diagnosing an underactive thyroid is that the symptoms are so general. 'In the early stages, patients are tired and a bit depressed, and a lot of the population have these symptoms.' says Dr Anthony Toft, a consultant endocrinologist at the Edinburgh Royal Infirmary.

He, too, believes that blood tests are the only accurate way to diagnose hypothyroidism. 'Blood tests are more accurate than our clinical judgement and before we had them and relied solely on clinical diagnosis many patients were unnecessarily started on courses of thyroxine.'

Despite his concerns, however, Dr. Toft, who is president of the British Thyroid Association, is about to embark on a study into whether patients with borderline TSH levels can benefit from thyroid hormones.

At the University of Sheffield, professor of medicine Tony Weetman is a firm believer in the value of blood tests. But he also points out that the signs of hypothyroidism can be so subtle that all doctors should have a low threshold for testing for the condition – as well as for repeated testing. 'If someone has one normal test, doctors should not conclude that they won't have thyroid disease in the future.' he says.

In April, writing in the *British Medical Journal,* Professor Weetman highlighted a potential problem with the current reference range used to assess TSH levels. The range was arrived at by assessing the blood of an apparently normal population – but because hypothyroidism is so common, people who are asymptomatic will have been included in the results.

Two months later, in the same journal, a group of doctors called for thyroxine to be offered as a trial treatment to patients with clinical symptoms of hypothyroidism, but whose biochemistry appeared normal – precisely what Diana Holmes has been calling for.

Dr Andrew Wright, a GP in Bolton, was one of the signatories. His interest arose because of the large number of chronic fatigue syndrome patients he was seeing who appeared to have some metabolic underactivity. 'One reason for this was thyroid deficiency and I began to realise there were some problems with thyroid testing. The reference range is too wide,' he says. 'Then I heard of work coming from America which showed that not only can patients be hypothyroid because of a thyroid gland problem, but also because other hormones – including melatonin and cortisol – are affecting thyroid function.' But Dr Wright says that British endocrinologists do not yet seem interested in this story.

At the Royal College of General Practitioners, honorary secretary Dr Bill Reith has been in correspondence with Mrs Holmes and has some sympathy for her views. 'There is the possibility that patients are being missed because hypothyroidism comes on gradually and individual patients present at differing stages in the development of their illness.'

Although he agrees that clinical symptoms must be taken into account as well as blood tests, he thinks that when patients present with the conundrum of having normal blood bio-chemistry, they should be referred to a specialist rather than be treated by their family doctor. Mrs Holmes has no arguments with this.

'All I want is for doctors to be less rigid in their interpretation of blood test results,' she says.

165

APPENDIX III

BRITISH MEDICAL JOURNAL
CORRRESPONDENCE

BMJ VOLUME 314: 14 JUNE 1997

Thyroxine should be tried in clinical hypothyroid but biochemically euthyroid patients

EDITOR—We wish to question present medical practice, which considers abnormal serum concentrations of free thyroxine and thyroid stimulating hormone — those outside the 95% reference interval — to indicate hypothyroidism but incorrectly considers 'normal' free thyroxine and thyroid stimulating hormone concentrations to negate this diagnosis. [1] It is unusual for doctors to start thyroxine replacement in clinically hypothyroid but biochemically euthyroid patients.

The free thyroxine and thyroid stimulating hormone concentrations in 80 patients considered to be hypothyroid on established criteria indicated that only five patients had free thyroxine concentrations (just) below the reference interval of 10-19 pmol/1 (values of 9.4, 9.8, 9.9, and 9.9 pmol/1 and only four patients had thyroid stimulating hormone values above the reference interval of 0.5-5.5mU/1 (values of 5.6, 8.4, 11.8 and 30.1 mU/1); moreover in these 80 patients the mean concentration of thyroid stimulating hormone was 2.2 (0.4) m/UI; both of these values lie well within the normal reference intervals. While we accept that there will be subjective variation in the evaluation of clinical diagnostic criteria and that the long term response to thyroid replacement is a prerequisite of our proposition, exclusion of hypothyroidism on the grounds of hormone concentrations measured in the laboratory seems wrong.

We contend that an incremental three month trial of thyroxine treatment in clinically hypothyroid but biochemically euthyroid patients is a safe and reasonable strategy. The dangers of

---

[1] Weetman AP. Hypothyroidism: screening and subclinical disease.*BMJ* 1997; 314:1175-78. (19 April).

osteoporosis and cardiac catastrophe — particularly during a three month trial — are sometimes quoted, but these worries are unfounded and condemn many patients to years of hypothyroidism with its pathological complications and poor quality of life. We urge that the question of clinical hypothyroidism in biochemically euthyroid patients should be subjected to a formal clinical trial.

Gordon R.B. Skinner *Clinical virologist*
Harborough Banks, Old Warwick Road, Lapworth, Warwickshire B94 6LD
R Thomas *General practitioner*
Old Road Surgery, Llanelli, Carmarthenshire SS2 6LQ
M Taylor *General practitioner*
9 East Street, Prittlewell, Southend on Sea, Essex SS2 6LQ
M Sellarajah *General practitioner*
115 Humberstone Road, Pype Hayes, Erdington B24 0PY
S Bolt *General practitioner*
Westcotes Health Centre, Leicester LE3 0LP
S Krett *General practitioner*
118 Station road, Hendon, London NN4 3FN
A Wright*General practitioner*
57 Chorley New Road, Bolton BL1 4QR

Trial of thyroxine treatment for biochemically euthyroid patients has been approved.

EDITOR—Skinner et al's suggestion that patients with symptoms of hypothyroidism and normal results of thyroid function tests might benefit from treatment with thyroxine [1] received considerable publicity in our local evening newspaper. As a result several patients were referred to our clinic.

Since they complained of a considerable reduction in their quality of life, which had not been helped by other measures, we decided that it was justifiable to try treating two of them with 100 ug thyroxine daily (after we explained the lack of scientific rationale and obtained their written consent). Much to our surprise, they both reported a considerable improvement in their conditions, while the result of thyroid function tests remained within the reference range; one of them returned to work after an absence of four years. Although this may well have been a placebo response, it should be noted that such patients are often given repeated course of antidepressants (at worst an expensive and dangerous placebo) without apparent effect.

While our present state of knowledge suggests that there is no scientific justification for this treatment, it is intellectually arrogant to assume that we know everything about the physiology of thyroid secretion and its controlling hormones or the pharmacological effects of exogeneous thyroxine. [2] In view of the lack of effective treatment for this group of patients, we believe that further investigation of the effect of thyroxine is justified, as Skinner et al proposed. We have now received approval from our local ethics committee for a double blind placebo controlled trial of thyroxine in patients with symptoms of hypothyroidism and normal results of thyroid function tests.

E H McLaren I *consultant physician*
C J Kelly *Specialist registrar in endocrinology*
M A Pollok *Principal biochemist*
Stobhill NHS Trust, Glasgow G21 3UW

---

[1] Giving thyroid hormones to clinically hypothyroid but biochemically euthyroid patients [letters] *BMJ* 1997;315;813-4 (27 September).
[2] Skinner GRB Thomas R, Taylor M, Sellaraja M, Bolt S, Krett S, et al. Thyroxine should be tried in clinically hypothyroid but biochemically euthyroid patients. *BMJ* 1997;314:1764 (14 June).

APPENDIX IV

EXAMPLES OF BLOOD TEST RESULTS FOR THYROID FUNCTION:

The reference ranges used against blood tests results vary. It depends which "assay pack" the laboratory has received. They should all be worked out on the same principle. The most usual thyroid function tests are: TSH, TT4, FT4, and FT3.

TSH.: Thyroid Stimulating Hormone comes from the pituitary to stimulate the thyroid gland into making more hormone. **TSH** rises when the thyroid is struggling. In your area the **TSH** reference range may be approx. 0.4 - 4.5.

Your result may be within the so-called normal range as shown in the figure below at 2.1 or 3.9, but your thyroid may still be struggling.*

	4.5	
	3.9	
	2.1	
	0.4	

* Remember you never had a blood test for thyroid function when you were well, there was no need – so ask the G.P., where is your BASE-LINE?

TT4 (Total T4.) Thyroid hormones bound to proteins. TT4 lowers when the thyroid is struggling.

In your area the TT4 reference range may be approx. 50 - 160.

Your result may be at 60, 70, 80, 90, 100 or 110 as shown in the figure below, yet still in the so-called normal range.*

	110	
	100	
	90	
	80	
	70	
	60	
	50	

*Again, ask the G.P. where is your BASE-LINE? You may need to be at the upper end of the normal reference range.

FT4: (Free T4.) Hormones not bound to protein. FT4 lowers when the thyroid is struggling.

In your area the FT4 reference range may be approx. 10 - 24.

Your result may be 11, 12, 13, 14 or 15 as shown in the figure below. You may function better if your result is at the upper end of the range.*

	24	
	15	
	14	
	13	
	12	
	11	
	10	

*Again where is your BASE-LINE?

FT3: (Free T3.) Hormones not bound to protein ready to be taken up by the cells.

Reference ranges approx: 3.5 - 6.5. Your result maybe 3.9 or 4.0 as shown in the figure below, but may need to be at the upper end of normal for you to function properly.

_____	**6.5**	_____
	4.0	
	3.9	
_____	**3.5**	_____

Again, the important question is where were your levels to start with?

Things to watch out for:

[1] The paragraph below is taken from the book - *Thyroid Disease: the Facts* by Dr. R.I. Bayliss and Dr. W.M. Turnbridge (Oxford University Press).

"Under certain circumstances, for example in pregnancy, or when taking oestrogens, or the contraceptive pill or certain other drugs, the amount of carrier protein is increased. This increases the T.T.4 level but does not make the subject hypothyroid because the free non-protein bound thyroxine remains normal."

In this instance it is better to carry out an F.T.4 blood test.

[2] According to Medicine International 1993 the Medicine Group of (Journals) Ltd. State, "T.S.H. levels are normal in approximately 50% of patients with hypothyroidism secondary to hypothalamic or pituitary disease but T.T.4 and F.T.4 are usually low."

Biochemists in the laboratory are refusing to carry out an F.T.4 blood test if the T.S.H. is normal. Why are they not in receipt of this important information? Neither biochemist nor G.P. had a base-line to work from, because the patient did not have a blood test carried out when they were well.

APPENDIX V

POEMS

Why Don't You Listen?

I am ill, but you just don't want to see,
The times I've told you what's happening to me,
    All the tests and the pain that I've gone through,
    Makes me angry, I start to despise you.

I have heard it all before – believe you me,
It's not all in my head as you would like it to be.
    Instead of shouting, bullying and having fits,
    Just LISTEN, don't pass me on to a psychiatrist.

You treat me as though I am stupid and thick
And then talk to me like I don't exist,
    Why don't you sit down and try to explain
    I am human – I've got a brain.

I can only tell you what it's like
This illness that makes me have no life.
    To walk, to run, to be able to think without pain,
    Just to get my old self back again.

If you don't know what's really wrong,
Why don't you say so, I am strong,
    I must confess that I'm baffled too,
    So let's work together and battle it through.

CAROLE WILLIAMS

Beautiful Memories Treasured Forever of My Late Wife, Hilda Patricia [1]

We sat by your bedside,
We held your hand with love,
We stroked your head with tenderness
And prayed to God above.

In tears we watched you fading
We watched you slip away,
You meant so very much to us
Much more than words can say.

I saw you suffer, heard you sigh
And all I could do was just stand by
When the time came I suffered too
You never deserved what you went through.

My heart still aches as I whisper Love
God bless you, Love, I miss you so.
A prayer, a tear, till the end of time
Missing you always forgetting you never
A bouquet of roses just for you
Sprinkled with teardrops instead of dew
Place in the centre a forget-me-not
To tell you, Pat, we haven't forgot.

We think of you with love today as we so often do.

If tears could build a staircase and memories make a lane
I'd walk straight up to heaven love and bring you home again.
So those of you who have a wife, love her while you may
For I would give my everything to see my Pat today.

In God's own time we will meet again.

DAVID TINSLEY

---

[1] When David telephoned to tell me about his wife Hilda, I was very distressed. Apparently Hilda had been found to be hypothyroid years ago. She was given one month's supply of thyroxine and after that no one followed up her case. She had been quite poorly with the condition and was not responsible for herself. She did not receive any medication for eighteen months after that. By January 1994, she was admitted to hospital with severe senile dementia and a grossly underactive thyroid. Hilda passed away. Her husband David Tinsley wrote this poem in remembrance of her.

173

Chronic M.E.

I'm at a loss for words to say,
What was said the other day?
　　I've been ill for a long time,
　　Now I feel I've committed a crime.

The doctors who should really care,
Don't understand, they just stare,
　　This horrid disease they can't make out,
　　Just makes me want to shout.

My eyes, my arms, my legs and head,
Make we want to stay in bed,
　　If I don't and do what they say,
　　I'm the one who has to pay.

I can't walk far on my own,
So use a wheel-chair with chaperone,
　　With my independence/dignity gone too
　　I'm told its caused by "yuppie 'flu".

Now here's the best that I've heard yet
From stupid people I've just met,
　　"It's a virus that can't be found
　　It doesn't last long it goes to ground."

We don't give care and mobility,
To those who question society,
　　There is no help that we can give,
So get out there and start to live.

CAROLE WILLIAMS

Barnes, Broda M.D. *Hypothyroidism and The Unsuspected Illness* New York, Harper & Row, 1976.

Bayliss Dr. R.I. and Tunbridge Dr. W.M. *Thyroid Disease the Facts,* Oxford University Press, 1991.

Gomez Dr. Joan, *Coping with Thyroid Problems,* Sheldon Press, 1994.

Hillson Dr,. Rowan, *Thyroid Disorders,* Optima 1991.

Mindell Earl, *The Vitamin Bible,* Arlington Books (Publishers) Ltd, London.

Pizzorno, Joseph, M.D. *Total Wellness* Prima Publishing, P.O. Box 1260BK, CA 95677, USA

Readers Digest, *Foods that harm Foods that Heal.*

Westcott Patsy, *Thyroid Problems,* Thorsons 1995.

Wilson, E. Denis M.D. *Wilson's Syndrome: The Miracle of Feeling Well,* Florida, Cornerstone Publications, Second Edition, 1993.

Campaign for Informed Consent i.e. for surgery and medication e.g. hysterectomies and HRT.

Mrs. S. McShane
19 St. Edward Gardens,
Eggbuckland,
Plymouth,
PL6 5PB